Fluid and Electrolytes
In Practice

Fluid and Electrolytes In Practice

HARRY STATLAND, M.D.

Associate in Medicine, University of Kansas School of Medicine; Consultant in Medicine, Veterans Administration Hospital, Kansas City, Missouri; Attending Physician, Menorah Medical Center, Kansas City, Missouri

J. B. LIPPINCOTT COMPANY

Philadelphia   Montreal

Library of Congress
Catalog Card Number
54-11529

PRINTED IN THE UNITED STATES OF AMERICA

TO MY PARENTS
IDA AND SAMUEL STATLAND

Preface

The material in this book was first presented as a series of lectures to undergraduate and postgraduate students at the University of Kansas School of Medicine, in 1950. It was at the request of many of these students that the notes have here been assembled, amplified and presented as a practical guide to fluid and electrolyte therapy.

In presenting the necessary chemistry and physiology, perhaps I have erred on the side of oversimplification, in order to keep the text intelligible to those practicing physicians who have long been removed from the basic sciences. While nothing has been sacrificed in accuracy or completeness by this, I have felt that it was justified in the interests of practicability. The physiologic principles upon which proper therapy is based have not been concentrated into any single chapter; rather, they are discussed at different points throughout the text where the discussion seemed to adapt itself to a logical explanation of the clinical picture and the management. For this reason frequent cross references are made in order to avoid repetition.

Part One presents the basic principles of fluid movements and the major abnormalities of volume, concentration and acid-base balance. In this section the management of the surgical patient has been stressed particularly. In Part Two the application to management of special diseases is discussed more fully. A thorough understanding of Part One is necessary in order to apply effectively the principles of management discussed in Part Two.

The volume of literature on this subject has become so great that it is impossible to mention all the excellent papers that have been published. Therefore, the bibliography includes only a representative selection of articles which either demonstrate certain important principles or have some clinical bearing on these principles. I have drawn heavily on the work of J. L. Gamble, J. P. Peters, D. C. Darrow and A. M. Butler, who have been the pioneers in this field. The more recent literature has been stressed particularly, in the bibliography.

I am especially indebted to Dr. Alexander Leaf at the Massachusetts General Hospital for his discussions and help in the early stages of preparation of this book. I am grateful to Dr. Jack Zellermayer, Dr. Sidney Rubin and Dr. Morris Statland for reading the manuscript and for their many suggestions. Miss Lois Brunner and Miss Rita Carr, medical technicians, were of great help in developing the fluid balance service and in the study of fluid problems in many patients. I wish also to thank Mrs. Angelika Howard and Mrs. Evelyn LeVine for their help in checking the bibliography, and Mrs. Mary Lou Stickel for typing the manuscript. The drawings were made by Miss Arlene Nichols.

H.S.

Contents

PART ONE

General Principles

PART TWO

Application to Special Conditions

Part One

GENERAL PRINCIPLES

CHAPTER ONE

Fluid Structure

ELECTROLYTES

By electrolytes we refer to those substances which, when placed in water, dissociate into charged particles called ions. Positively charged ions are spoken of as **cations**, and in the blood they are Na^+, K^+, Ca^{++} and Mg^{++}. The negatively charged ions, called **anions**, are Cl^-, PO^{--}, HCO_3^-, organic acids and proteins. Other substances, such as urea and glucose, are also present in blood serum, but since they have no electric charges and do not dissociate into charged particles they are not electrolytes.

CHEMICAL EQUIVALENTS

In studying the alterations in blood chemistries and their concentration we are not concerned with how much the ions weigh (mg. %), but rather with how many ions there are (mEq./L.). The milliequivalent system of terminology is an important tool in the understanding of this subject and it is virtually impossible to follow electrolyte shifts when they are expressed as milligrams per cent. If the reader will forgive a simple but point-making analogy, one might compare this to the hostess making up her list of guests to a dance. She does not invite 1,000 pounds of girls for 1,000 pounds of boys. Rather, she is interested in how many of each, and, regardless of difference in weights, the number of individual males and females (anions and cations) must be equal.

As an example, since the atomic weight of sodium is 23, 23 Gm. of sodium is one equivalent of sodium, chemically speaking. Expressing this in milligrams, rather than grams, and in milliequivalents, instead of equivalents, therefore:

> 23 mg. of sodium is 1 milliequivalent
> 46 mg. of sodium is 2 mEq.
> 69 mg. of sodium is 3 mEq., and so on.

The atomic weight of chlorine, on the other hand, is 35. Therefore, 35 Gm. of chlorine is one chemical equivalent, and 35 Gm. of chlorine combines equally with only 23 Gm. of sodium. Expressed in milligrams then:

> 35 mg. of chlorine is 1 mEq.
> 70 mg. of chlorine is 2 mEq.
> 105 mg. of chlorine is 3 mEq., and so on.

It is apparent then that dividing the number of milligrams of a monovalent substance by its atomic weight gives the number of combining particles or milliequivalents. Milligrams are ordinarily reported in terms of 100 cc. of solution and milliequivalents are reported in terms of 1,000 cc. of solution so we have to multiply by 10 in converting from milligrams to milliequivalent terminology.

So far we have discussed ions which have a valence of 1, that is, ions, which have a single electric charge. Since each atom of a bivalent substance has 2 charges, it can combine with 2 monovalent ions. The atomic weight of such a substance therefore represents 2 chemical equivalents. The atomic weight of calcium is 40. Therefore, 40 mg. of calcium is 2 mEq., since this amount would combine with 2 mEq. of Cl^-, which is monovalent. The rule then becomes: To convert mg. % to mEq./L.:

$$\frac{mg.\%}{atomic\ wt.} \times 10 \times valence = mEq./L.$$

TABLE 1. CONVERSION OF THE MORE COMMONLY USED
ELECTROLYTES FROM MG.% TO MEQ./L.

Na^+	mg.% x 10 ÷ 23	= mEq./L.
K^+	mg.% x 10 ÷ 39	= mEq./L.
Cl^-	mg.% x 10 ÷ 35	= mEq./L.
Ca^{++}	mg.% x 10 ÷ 40 x 2	= mEq./L.
Mg^{++}	mg.% x 10 ÷ 24 x 2	= mEq./L.
CO_2 Vol.%	÷ 2.22	= mEq./L.

Table 1 shows the conversion of the commonest electrolytes from mg.% to mEq./L. Note that carbon dioxide combining power is converted to milliequivalents by dividing volume per cent by 2.22.

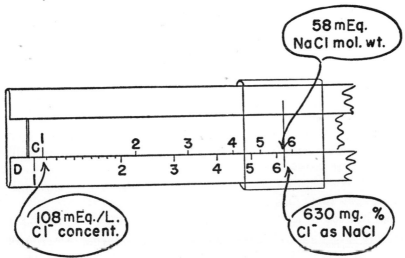

FIG. 1. Slide rule conversion of milligram per cent to milli-equivalents per liter. Serum chloride, expressed as sodium chloride (NaCl) in mg. %, may be converted to mEq./L. by one setting on the slide rule. The determination in mg. % is set under 58 (molecular weight of NaCl), and the Index 1 indicates the reading of chloride (Cl) in mEq./L.

Until hospitals begin to use the milliequivalent system in reporting serum electrolytes, it will be necessary for the physician to make quick conversions. For this purpose a celluloid pocket slide rule is most helpful. As shown in Figure 1, the slide rule will convert milligrams per cent of chloride, reported as sodium chloride, to milliequivalents per liter by a single setting. One should make certain however that the chlorides are measured in serum and not in whole blood since the two values are appreciably different. For electrolyte balance purposes, blood chemistries are of relatively little value compared to serum chemistries, since the determinations may be altered by the degree of anemia or by hemoconcentration. This is true because of the marked difference of chemical values in the serum as compared to blood cells.

OSMOTIC EFFECTS

If two different solutions are separated by a membrane impermeable to the dissolved substances, there will occur a shift of fluid through the membrane from the least concentrated to the more concentrated solution, until the solutions are of equal concentration. This is termed osmosis and the dissolved substances are said to exert an osmotic force in causing the fluid shift. The magnitude of this force is dependent upon the number of particles dissolved and not upon their weights or valences. Thus 10 atoms of sodium have the same osmotic force as 10 atoms of calcium or 10 molecules of protein, in spite of the differences in valence and weight. Sodium, therefore, exerts a more potent osmotic force than the same weight of protein since there are so many more molecules of sodium than protein in a given weight of both substances. The term milliosmole refers to this osmotic effect of a substance. One mEq. of sodium (23 mg.) exerts 1 mOsm. of pressure. However, 2 mEq. of calcium (40 mg.) also exerts only 1 mOsm. of pressure. Bivalent atoms have a chemical equivalence of 2 but the osmotic force of only 1 particle. Therefore:

$$\frac{mg. \%}{atomic\ wt.} \times 10 = mOsm./L.$$

By way of review, normal saline has 150 mEq. of sodium. How many milliequivalents of chloride in this solution? The answer is 150 mEq. of chloride, since there is 1 atom of chloride for each atom of sodium. How many milliosmoles of sodium chloride in this solution? The answer would be 300, since there are 150 mOsm. each of sodium and chloride. The osmotic force of this solution would be the effect of both ions combined. Again, if a solution of calcium chloride, $CaCl_2$, has 150 mEq. of chloride, how many milliequivalents of calcium has it? The answer is 150 mEq. of calcium. How many milliosmoles of calcium? There are 75 mOsm. How many milliosmoles of $CaCl_2$? The answer is 225 mOsm. of $CaCl_2$ which represents the total of 150 of chloride and 75 of calcium.

FLUID COMPARTMENTS OF THE BODY

In planning therapy for the depleted patient a knowledge of the volumes normally present in the various fluid compartments is of great value and well worth remembering. Since the chemical make-up of fluid is fairly constant, one can often estimate the quantity of electrolyte loss from each compartment if the total fluid loss is known. Loss of 1 L. of cell fluid, for example, will carry with it its dissolved electrolytes and some of the protein.

The body fluids are divided into two major compartments (Fig. 2) and the volumes, expressed as a fraction of the total body weight, are as follows:

Total body fluid.............60 per cent of body weight
Cellular fluid
   compartment (CF)........40 per cent of body weight
Extracellular fluid
   compartment (EF)........20 per cent of body weight

The total fluid of the body varies within fairly wide limits depending upon the amount of fatty tissue, which has less water, and of muscular tissue ("lean body mass") which has a greater percentage of water. More accurately speaking the average figure would be about 56 per cent of body weight. In

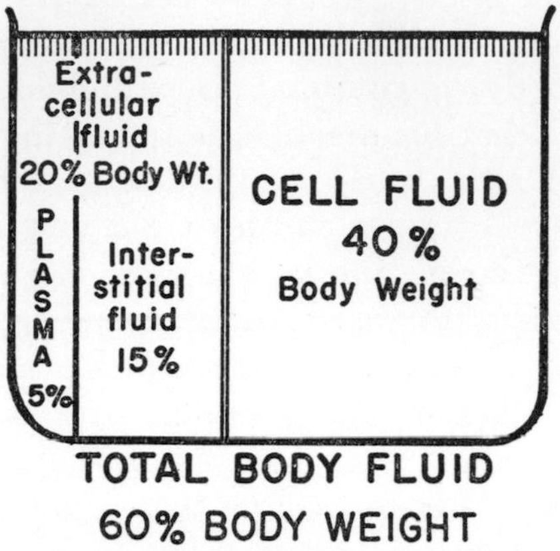

Extra-
cellular
fluid
20% Body Wt.

CELL FLUID
40%
Body Weight

P
L
A
S
M
A
5%

Inter-
stitial
fluid
15%

TOTAL BODY FLUID
60% BODY WEIGHT

Fig. 2. Fluid compartments of the body. The total body fluid is about 60 per cent of the body weight, varying with the amount of fat tissue present. For practical purposes of therapy, there are two major divisions of this fluid, (A) the cellular fluid compartment, 40 per cent of the body weight, and (B) the extracellular fluid compartment, 20 per cent of the body weight. The latter is made up of the plasma (5 per cent b.w.) and interstitial fluid (15 per cent b.w.). The capillary wall which separates these two is a "rapid membrane" as to transport of electrolytes across it, and the interstitial fluid, in effect, becomes a reservoir for the blood plasma. The cell wall, however, is a "slow membrane" and metabolic processes within the cell govern the movement of electrolytes crossing this barrier.

women the average total body fluid is about 52 per cent of body weight, and in men, about 60 per cent.

The extracellular fluid may be divided into the plasma fluid (5 per cent of body weight) and interstitial fluid (15 per cent of body weight), but for practical purposes they may be considered together as a single compartment. More accurately again, the extracellular compartment is about 16 per cent of body weight. Although the percentages in the above table have been idealized to their nearest round figures, they are accurate enough for clinical purposes and make computation for replacement therapy more simple. The value of being familiar with the major compartments can be illustrated in the following example. Let us assume that a sick individual has lost, over a period of days, about 2,100 cc. of body fluids and demonstrates clinically the picture of primary water dehydration. Since the chemical structure of the two major compartments is quite different, the repair solutions must take into account this difference. In this patient one might safely estimate that one third ($\frac{2}{6}$) of 2,100, or 700 cc., was derived from the extracellular fluid and two thirds ($\frac{4}{6}$) of 2,100, or 1,400 cc., from the cellular fluid. The replacement solution for this patient should follow this proportion also, i.e., one third to replace the loss of extracellular fluid and two thirds to replace the cellular fluid loss with their different chemical structures.

Although considerable advantage would be gained if measurement of the various compartments were clinically feasible, the methods available to date are still too complex for routine use. Measurement of the extracellular space is most accurately determined by the inulin method, although sodium thiocyanate has been widely used. The total body water may be measured using deuterium oxide (heavy water), and the difference between these two values would represent the volume of intracellular fluid. Blood and plasma volume can be determined by Evans' Blue dye and also by red blood cells labeled with radioactive phosphorous (P^{32}). It is beyond our scope to present the methods involved in these determinations and the reader is referred to the original descriptions.

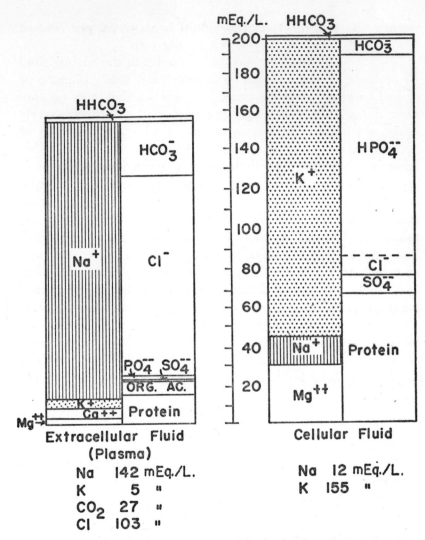

FIG. 3. Chemical composition of body fluids. The height of the columns and of the individual electrolytes represent the concentration in mEq./L. of fluid. The concentration of substance in the plasma is not synonymous with the quantity. In dehydration, for example, loss of sodium (Na^+) will diminish its total amount in the plasma, but its concentration will be elevated since water is lost in proportionately greater amounts. The preponderance of sodium in the extracellular compartment and of potassium (K^+) in the cellular compartment is evident. (Modified from Gamble)

CHEMICAL STRUCTURE OF FLUIDS

In current medical literature some confusion has arisen in the meaning of the terms "base" and "acid." It is incorrect to use these to mean cations and anions, respectively, in pure chemical terminology. However, it has become so widely accepted through common usage in clinical medicine that we shall continue to use "base" for cation and "acid" for anion throughout this volume.

Extracellular Fluid

Let us examine first the composition of the EF (Fig. 3). For all practical purposes plasma and interstitial fluid can be considered to be identical in chemical structure. It will be seen that the total of cations equals the total of the anions since there must be a negatively charged ion for every positive ion. A change in concentration of the cations will produce a change in concentration of anions and vice versa. The pre-

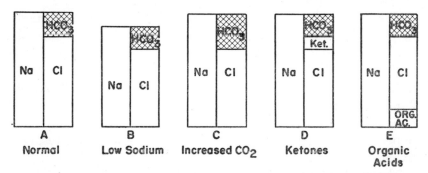

Fig. 4. Acid-base equivalance of extracellular fluid. (A) The total number of anion molecules must equal the number of cation molecules. If a patient were found to have a *low serum chloride*, one of the following compensatory changes would have to be present also: (B) The total base (sodium [Na] primarily) would be decreased; (C) Or, if the sodium was of normal concentration, the CO_2 combining power would be increased; (D) Or ketonic acids would be present as in starvation or diabetes; (E) Or there would be increased organic acids as in uremia. Likewise, if a low sodium were found, the concomitant findings would have to be decreased chloride (Cl), decreased CO_2 combining power or both.

dominant cation present is sodium which makes up more than 90 per cent of the total base at a concentration of 142 mEq./L. Because of its predominant quantity, any appreciable change in total base really represents a change in sodium. This, plus the fact that sodium does not easily cross the cell wall membrane, gives it the primary role in controlling distribution of water throughout the body, as will be shown. It is this function of sodium which makes it so important in fluid balance. The concentration of sodium in the serum is carefully controlled by nerve receptors in the hypothalamus which are sensitive to changes in tonicity (concentration) of the blood. A drop in concentration of serum sodium will initiate a loss of fluid in an attempt to re-establish the normal concentration. On the other hand, an increase in sodium concentration stimulates water retention, diluting it back to its normal level. Alterations in sodium concentration, by causing water retention or loss, can in this way produce profound clinical effects in markedly influencing blood volume.

The other cations Ca^{++}, Mg^{++} and K^+, although important in physiology, have little, if any, effect on blood volume or fluid shifts. Small variations in their concentrations produce profound clinical effects. Normally K^+ is present in concentrations of about 5 mEq./L. and may cause death at levels of 2 mEq./L. or 10 mEq./L. Ca^{++} which is present in concentrations of about 5 mEq./L., will produce tetany or symptoms of hypercalcemia at levels of 3.5 mEq./L. or 7 mEq./L., respectively.

The predominant anions are chloride and bicarbonate. Their combined concentrations depend in large part on the concentration of total base (or sodium). They increase or decrease depending on sodium loss or gain (Fig. 4). The relation of chloride to bicarbonate depends upon factors influencing acid-base balance and these will be discussed at length in another chapter. Under normal conditions, the sum of chloride and bicarbonate equals the concentration of sodium minus 12 mEq. This applies only if there are no complicating factors such as ketosis, renal impairment or hemoconcentration. Therefore, one is not justified in using serum chloride and CO_2 combining power in lieu of serum sodium in many clinical states.

The remaining anions are organic acids (lactic and citric) and proteins. It is the difference in protein concentration between plasma and interstitial fluid that permits normal circulation of fluid from the capillary to the tissue spaces. In the presence of hemoconcentration, the elevation of protein concentration helps to maintain blood volume by drawing in fluid from the interstitial fluid.

CELLULAR FLUID

In examination of the composition of CF (Fig. 3), one is immediately struck by the marked dissimilarity between this and EF. The predominant cation here is potassium, with a concentration of about 150 mEq./L. It is present both as free ionic potassium in the cell fluid and combined with protein, as part of the protein molecule. Because of this latter fact there is a constant relationship between potassium and nitrogen excretion in the urine under conditions of normal metabolism. If one compares the great difference in concentration of this electrolyte within and outside the cell, and also takes into consideration the normal daily intake and output of 50 mEq., it is apparent that the serum potassium level of 5 mEq./L. in no way reflects the large turnover of this electrolyte. Potassium is involved in energy metabolism during the utilization of oxygen and glucose in the cell. It is for this reason, apparently, that potassium does not move into the cell in the absence of adequate supplies of glucose and insulin or if anoxemia exists. In the presence of cell dehydration or if metabolism is excessive, as with physical exertion and exercise, the liberation of potassium from its relatively high cellular concentration produces, in effect, a flooding of the blood plasma with the dislodged potassium. Under these conditions the levels of serum potassium may become elevated until potassium is excreted by the kidney. During dehydration, however, urine volume is apt to be low and potassium may be retained in the serum, even though there are large deficits within the cell.

While the concentration of potassium in the red blood cells roughly parallels the changes in the muscle cells, there is not general agreement that one can accurately use blood cell potassium determinations to reflect general body cell potassium levels. The difference in acid-base shifts, oxygenation and metabolic turnover, all of which may influence cell potassium concentration, are obviously different in blood cells and other tissues.

It was formerly believed that sodium never crossed the cell membrane, but recent work has indicated that there is approximately 12 mEq. of sodium within the cell, and that this plays an important role in variations of acid-base balance. It will be noted that this amount of sodium is about one half the concentration of bicarbonate outside the cell, but in view of the relatively large amount of CF as compared to EF, the total amount of sodium within the cell represents an appreciable amount in the body and is about equal to the total amount of extracellular bicarbonate. Generally speaking, there tends to be a reciprocal relationship between the amount of sodium and potassium in the cell fluids, an increase in one bringing about a decrease in the other. This does not represent simply a quantitative exchange of one ion for the other but is the result of cellular metabolic adjustments which will be discussed more fully later. Sodium is found in bone in considerably higher concentration than in other tissues. While the greater part is fixed, a fraction of this may be readily mobilized and it is believed that it may play an important role in the emergencies of acute bodily stress.

After potassium, magnesium is the most abundant cation in the cell, at a concentration of about 28 mEq./L. Like potassium, it is involved in energy transfer mechanisms and its movements into and out of the cell are, therefore, the result of metabolic processes rather than simple diffusion. Its full role in the causation of abnormal clinical states is only beginning to be understood.

Phosphate is the anion present in the cell in greatest concentration and this is involved in many of the energy transferring reactions and in the utilization of glucose. Small amounts of chloride have also been shown to be present within the cell, but the exact significance of this in clinical states is not yet understood.

CHAPTER TWO

Movement of Fluids in the Body

In the consideration of abnormal fluid movements within the body we must visualize two main forces as being ultimately involved. These are the hemodynamic forces of the blood and lymph circulation, and the shift resulting from change in concentrations of electrolytes and proteins in the various fluid compartments.

FLUID TRANSPORT THROUGH VESSELS

As shown by Starling, the normal movement of fluids through the capillary wall into the tissues depends on the force of the hydrostatic pressure at both the arterial and venous ends of the capillary, which tends to drive fluid out of the vessel (Fig. 5). On the other hand, the osmotic pressure exerted by the protein of the plasma exerts forces drawing fluid back into the capillary. The direction of movement of fluid depends on the resultants of these opposing forces. The hydrostatic force is greater than the osmotic force at the arterial end of the capillary and so fluid moves out of the vessel, leaving a more concentrated blood. The osmotic force is greater than the hydrostatic force at the venous end of the capillary and fluid therefore re-enters the capillary here. Fluid movement is also influenced by the tissue tension, so that edema is more apt to occur in the loose areolar tissue of the periorbital and genital areas. The lymphatics also play a role by removing excess proteins and fluid from the interstitial tissue, returning it to the venous circulation. Interference with lymphatic circulation causes an increase in tissue protein and may lead to localized areas of edema where the normal lymphatic flow is impeded.

In a patient presenting himself with edema, one therefore has to take into consideration low plasma protein concentration, such as occurs in nephrosis, cirrhosis or malnutrition; thrombophlebitis, or venous obstruction, which increases the venous hydrostatic pressure; and lymphatic block by either pressure or inflammatory change. In acute glomerulonephritis, the cause of edema has been attributed by many to seepage

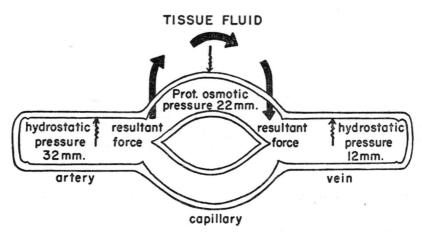

FIG. 5. Factors normally causing exchange of fluid across the capillaries. The forces which cause fluid to move in or out of the capillary are the resultants of osmotic pressure of proteins drawing fluid in, and hydrostatic pressure which pushes fluid out. The sum of these forces causes fluid to move *out* of the arterial end of the capillary and *in* at the venous end. Lymphatic flow and tissue tension also play a role. Since electrolyte concentrations in plasma and interstitial fluid are nearly identical, these have no influence on fluid circulation normally.

of plasma across the damaged capillary wall throughout the body, although cardiac failure with sodium retention may also be responsible. A combination of several of the above factors might produce edema, where the changes in any one alone would not be sufficient to cause it. A minor increase in venous pressure might cause considerable edema if, in addition, the blood proteins were appreciably lowered. For example, the ascites of cirrhosis may be due to the combination of obstruction in the portal veins and low serum protein as well as the loose structure of peritoneal surfaces. Changes in concentration of electrolytes on either side of the capillary wall will cause shifts of fluid which are unrelated to the above factors; the two processes may augment or decrease each other. Shifts of electrolytes may thus take place against the current of normal fluid circulation.

KIDNEY AND HORMONAL REGULATION

Since the intake of both water and electrolytes may vary in quantity within wide limits, it becomes the kidneys' function to regulate the excretion of these materials to conform with the intake and with the loss which may be occurring by other routes. Abnormal renal function, by either retaining too much or by losing too much, can seriously upset fluid or electrolyte balance.

Primarily, the formation of urine depends upon proper delivery of the fluid to the kidney. Defects of the transporting system such as occur in hemorrhage, shock, dehydration or extensive burns, all of which divert the fluids or blood flow from the kidneys, will not permit the kidney to exercise properly its control over excretion. The glomerular filtrate is formed as the result of a hydrostatic pressure in the glomerulus which exceeds the combined protein osmotic pull and the intraglomerular tissue tension by about 20 mm. of mercury. It is identical in composition to the plasma except for its protein content. In shock, or in any condition causing diminished renal flow, the effective filtration pressure is lessened and the volume of filtrate (normally about 180 L. daily), and, therefore, the amount of solutes, are diminished. Of this large volume of filtrate, about 85 per cent is reabsorbed by the proximal convoluted tubules and along with it about the same percentage of sodium.

The disposition of the remaining 15 per cent of the glomerular filtrate (about 27 L.) is dependent on the complex reabsorptive and secretory function of the distal tubules. Here, the kidneys need to reabsorb selectively different proportions of electrolytes and water, as well as other substances, so the resulting urine will be of either greater or less concentration than the protein-free plasma filtrate. This is influenced, to some degree, by the amount of water available and by the amount of waste to be excreted. In addition to reabsorption, the tubules also have a secretory function for disposing of some electrolytes, and also play the most important role in the regulation of the pH of blood. These various functions are all discussed in greater detail in later chapters.

CONTROL OF BLOOD OSMOLARITY

While a discussion of hormonal control of fluid might be considered academic, there are many situations in which an understanding of these mechanisms helps in the management of the patient. Forgetting for the moment the adjustment of acid-base balance, the body is confronted with two major problems in regulating the excretion of water and salt. One is *control of osmolarity* (solute concentration), and the other is *control of blood volume.*

The first of these involves an unknown control mechanism which sets the body's osmolarity at the level produced by 142 mEq./L. of sodium, rather than at some other level. This control organ has been called the "osmostat." The level of concentration dictated by the osmostat is maintained by cells believed to have been demonstrated by Verney in the supraoptic nucleus of the hypothalamus, which are known as "osmoreceptors," and which are sensitive to any variation from the established osmolarity. These cells control release of antidiuretic hormone (ADH) from the posterior pituitary. This hormone acts on Henle's loop in the kidney causing more water to be absorbed, forming a more concentrated urine.

The ADH plays a very important part in the renal control of water loss. If one takes a drink of water, the dilution of blood so produced inhibits the osmoreceptors and less ADH is released. Water reabsorption in the kidney tubules slows and a more dilute urine results. Conversely, lack of water or dehydration causes a more concentrated blood, ADH is released, water is reabsorbed in the tubules and the urine becomes more concentrated. The ability of the ADH to cause reabsorption of water is not unlimited, and urinary wastes (including sodium) will increase urine volume in spite of ADH action. It is doubtful, therefore, that edema could be caused by too much posterior pituitary hormone.

Clinical situations have been described in which the osmostat seems to be set at a lower level of osmolarity than is normally found. In a series of patients in whom malnutrition seemed to be the common factor to all, serum sodium levels were found to be considerably lowered, and yet there were none of the severe symptoms of salt depletion that one might have expected. Administration of extra salt to such individuals would merely be followed by increased salt excretion in the urine or, if this did not occur and the salt was retained, water would also be retained with resulting edema. On the other hand, in certain intracranial lesions involving the hypothalamus and frontal lobes, increased sodium concentrations are found without concomitant intracellular dehydration, apparently representing an abnormality in which the osmostat is set at higher osmolarity. Other clinical states with hypernatremia have not been described except that which occurs in primary water dehydration.

Absence of antidiuretic hormone gives rise to diabetes insipidus, in which the urine is very dilute and may exceed 15 L. in a day. Inability to concentrate under conditions of dehydration is diagnostic of this condition. Administration of posterior pituitary extract promptly corrects the defect; this being the basis of treatment for the condition. A functional diabetes insipidus has been described under conditions of emotional stress or after prolonged, excessive water-drinking. In the latter condition, chronic inhibition of ADH results in polyuria and exaggerated thirst. Likewise, inhibition of ADH production has been attributed to alcohol ingestion, negative pressure breathing and following exposure to cold, accounting for the polyuria seen in these clinical states.

CONTROL OF BLOOD VOLUME

The second major problem in water and salt regulation is that of maintenance of blood volume, but the site of this control is less well understood. Wherever the volume receptors are, they respond to a drop in blood volume by secreting the mineral hormones (desoxycorticosterone-like) of the adrenal cortex. These act on the distal convoluted tubules of the kidney to cause increased sodium reabsorption, and since a proportionate amount of water will also be reabsorbed, the blood volume is thereby increased. There is a limit however to the amount of sodium which will be reabsorbed and in the presence of normal adrenal function, when the blood has been restored to its usual volume, sodium reabsorption ceases in spite of increased amounts of mineral hormone. In the adrenalectomized or addisonian patient, however, this upper limitation seems to be lacking and edema may be produced by giving too much desoxycorticosterone. In the early stages of sodium loss, a water diuresis occurs to preserve the normal tonicity of blood serum, but as the blood volume drops, sodium excretion in the urine becomes negligible. If sodium continues to be lost from other routes (intestine, sweat), water is retained to maintain blood volume, despite the drop in concentration of sodium. The control of blood volume thus seems to have priority over control of concentration. The importance of this can be readily understood. Depletion of sodium leads to shocklike states, but this would be a much more frequent occurrence, if volume were not maintained regardless of drop in osmolarity. Besides this normal control of sodium loss, other steroid hormones may also cause increased sodium reabsorption, and these may produce abnormal amounts of sodium retention when given in excess.

In primary water loss with a drop in blood volume, sodium reabsorption is more complete and the plasma concentration of sodium increases. By excreting less sodium in the urine, water is conserved. This sparing action for water is aided by the antidiuresis resulting from the hypertonicity (stimulation of ADH release). Drop in blood volume due to hemorrhage or shock also initiates this sodium-conserving reaction, which has been called the "dehydration reaction."

Insufficient adrenal control, however, as found in destruction of the adrenal cortex, leads to the clinical picture of Addison's disease in which the kidneys are unable to retain sodium—the ultimate picture is, in large part, one of salt depletion. The use of desoxycorticosterone specifically corrects this feature of the disease, so that salt excretion abates. In the absence of the other adrenal cortical hormones, excess of DCA may cause edema from too much sodium retention.

Actually, the mechanisms for control of volume and osmolarity are not as simple as this discussion may make it appear. Clinical states in which ADH seems to function in the presence of low sodium, and in which salt is retained in spite of overexpanded extracellular volume are not uncommon and will be described more fully in later chapters (Chaps. 10 and 11).

FLUID MOVEMENTS AND CONCENTRATION CHANGES

EFFECTS OF SODIUM CONCENTRATION

The great importance of sodium in maintaining blood volume has already been pointed out, and because of its unique position in controlling osmotic relationships in all body fluids, alteration of its concentration in the plasma produces marked effects on the body. The experiments of Darrow and Yannet demonstrated these changes. Let us assume, for the purposes of this discussion, a simple organism consisting only of a cellular and extracellular compartment, with no circulating blood system or renal apparatus to make adjustments. If sodium chloride is added to the EF without added water, (Fig. 6), this fluid becomes hypertonic in comparison to the cell fluid. The osmotic force so created causes water to leave the more dilute cell fluid and enter the EF compartment. The CF thus becomes more concentrated, while the EF becomes diluted

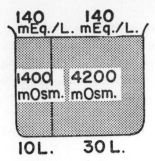

140 mEq./L.   140 mEq./L.

1400 mOsm.   4200 mOsm.

10 L.   30 L.

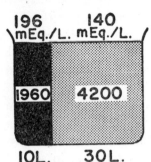

196 mEq./L.   140 mEq./L.

1960   4200

10 L.   30 L.

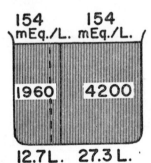

154 mEq./L.   154 mEq./L.

1960   4200

12.7 L.   27.3 L.

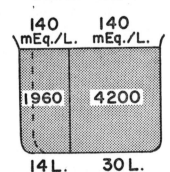

140 mEq./L.   140 mEq./L.

1960   4200

14 L.   30 L.

Fig. 6. Fluid shifts resulting from increasing the sodium concentration. This represents the extracellular fluid (EF) and cellular fluid (CF) compartments of 10 and 30 L. respectively. Being in osmotic balance, they both have sodium concentrations of 140 mEq./L. The total milliequivalents (or milliosmoles, to denote their osmotic activity) in the extracellular fluid is 1,400 (10 L. at 140 mEq./L.). In the cell fluid it is 4,200 mOsm. (30 L. at 140 mEq./L.)

Here 560 mOsm. were added to the EF (*left*). The total milliosmoles here are now increased by that amount. The concentration of sodium is now 196 mEq./L. This is hypertonic as compared to the CF.

Water begins to shift from CF (*right*) to the EF compartment until osmotic equilibrium is reached and both have concentrations of 154 mEq./L., but note that the EF is now expanded and the CF is now contracted. The added sodium is still in the extracellular fluid compartment (1,960 mOsm.), but by increasing the extracellular fluid volume the concentration has now been equalized in the two compartments. There has been no movement of electrolytes into or out of the cells.

To correct the elevated sodium concentration back to its original level of 140 mEq./L., 4 L. of water are added (the amount required to make the original 560 mEq. of sodium equal to 140 mEq./L.) and the original concentration is restored. Note that all the extra fluid and sodium is still in the EF (*left*) which is now expanded by the whole 4 L., and none of which has gone into the cell. (Data from Peters) with the result that there is equal concentration in both compartments. The total fluid in the organism has not changed, but the EF has expanded at the expense of the CF. Although the added sodium remains in the EF compartment, its osmotic effect has been exerted on all fluid compartments. Therefore, in raising the concentration of sodium in EF to a desired level, enough sodium needs to be added to raise the concentration

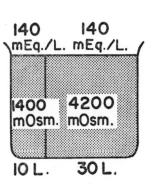

Fig. 7. Fluid shifts resulting from decreasing sodium concentration. This represents the extracellular fluid (EF) and cellular fluid (CF) compartments as in the previous figure.

Here 560 mEq. of sodium have been removed from the EF (*left*) leaving 840 mOsm., which in 10 L. gives a concentration of 84 mEq./L. The EF is now hypotonic as compared to the CF.

The fluid now begins to shift from the EF to the CF compartment until osmotic equilibrium is reached and both have a concentration of 126 mEq./L. Note that the EF is now contracted to 6.7 L. and the CF expanded to 33.3 L. The number of milliosmoles of sodium in the two compartments does not change; only the water has shifted equalizing the concentrations of electrolytes. (Data from Peters.)

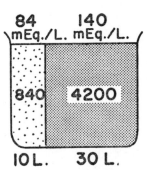

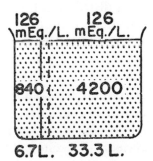

to this same level in all fluids in the body (even though the added sodium will remain extracellularly). If, in an individual, an increase in sodium concentration in the EF results from water loss, the same sequence of events occurs, with shift of fluid from the cellular to the extracellular compartments. Loss of water alone, therefore, causes depletion of fluid in all compartments.

If proportionate quantities of sodium and water (making a concentration of 140 mEq./L.) were added to the EF, the ultimate effect is to merely increase the volume of this compartment without changing the concentration of sodium (Fig. 6D). This is true because the added water and sodium is isotonic, and, therefore, causes no osmotic shift of fluid. Of course, this is strictly true only in a simple, closed system of fluids. In the presence of good cardiac function and normal kidneys, the expanded volume of the EF compartment would be corrected *in time* by excretion of the excess water and salt. In the presence of cardiac decompensation or poor kidney function, such an excess of volume might be difficult to remove because of impaired ability to excrete sodium.

If sodium chloride is removed from the EF (Fig. 7), the fluid becomes hypotonic in comparison to the CF. The osmotic effect is to cause fluid to leave the more dilute EF compartment and shift into the relatively more concentrated CF, resulting in equal concentration in both compartments. The EF becomes more concentrated and the cellular fluid more dilute. Here again the total fluid within the system has not changed, but the cellular fluid has been expanded at the expense of the EF. The osmotic effect (of removing the sodium from the EF) has been distributed through the total fluid of the system. Loss of salt alone from the EF, therefore, causes a depletion of fluid in the EF and an overhydration of cells.

To correct the lowered concentration of sodium produced by this experiment, it would not suffice to add only the amount of sodium deficient in the EF (that is 14 mEq. x 6.7 L.). To raise the concentration of sodium in EF by 14 mEq., the osmotic concentration must be raised in the total fluid of the system. Therefore, 14 mEq. x 40 L., or 560 mEq., would be required. Adding this amount of sodium in the form of 4 L. of isotonic saline would *not* correct the deficiency, since the effect produced in Figure 6D would then be obtained. That is, 4 L. at 126 mEq./L. would merely expand the EF compartment and only the remaining 14 mEq./L. (56 mEq., total) would be free to raise the concentration. This amount would be negligible. A beneficial clinical effect would be gained, however, since it would increase the volume of the EF.

In the presence of a low extracellular sodium concentration in a patient, one could, in time, correct sodium deficiency by giving normal saline, providing there was good cardiac and renal function so that the excess water given would be eliminated. In the presence of cardiac decompensation or renal impairment, the volume of fluid required to correct a sodium deficiency by using normal saline would be enough to precipitate acute failure.

POTASSIUM EFFECTS

Up to this point, we have placed considerable emphasis on the role of sodium in the osmolarity of all body fluids, and this will be the basis for subsequent discussions. However, it is well to call attention to the fact that there is some question about the truth of this long established concept. It has been suggested that the intracellular fluid osmolarity may be dependent on other factors as well. The intracellular base is visualized as being in both an ionic or osmotically effective state, and in a bound or osmotically inactive form. With certain metabolic changes, release of the bound electrolyte adds to the osmotic force intracellularly. Potassium, being the preponderant cellular cation, may play a role in the fluid movement by its metabolic functions and by its shifts into and out of the cell. The apparent inability of the kidneys to conserve potassium may influence cellular water, in that excretion of the dislodged potassium frees the water carried out of the cell with it, for use in the EF compartment. Increased metabolism, exertion, stress and adrenal hormones may thus be factors in altering intracellular osmolarity, potassium loss and cellular dehydration.

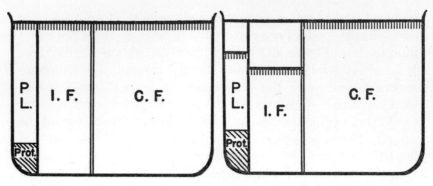

FIG. 8. The effect of protein on electrolyte shifts. (*Left*) The normal fluid compartments. (*Right*) Fluid has been lost from the plasma (PL.) causing hemoconcentration, thereby raising the protein concentration. The effect of this is to cause movement of sodium, chloride and water into the plasma compartment from the interstitial fluid (I.F.) (Donnan's equilibrium). Thus, the blood volume tends to stay up in dehydration at the expense of interstitial fluid.

PROTEIN CONCENTRATION EFFECTS

The presence of protein in the plasma, in amounts greater than that in interstitial fluid, also influences fluid shifts in a manner that tends to preserve blood volume (Fig. 8). Increasing the osmotic pressure of the plasma by hemoconcentration from either fluid loss or salt depletion, as in the above experiments, causes sodium, chloride and fluid to shift from the interstitial fluid to the plasma.

CHAPTER THREE

Intake, Output and Variations

Since there is no depot or reserve supply of fluid in the body as there is for other metabolic substances such as fat, glycogen, etc., failure to supply adequate amounts of fluid daily will result in its being drawn from the tissues in order to meet the continuous requirements of excretion. The fluid accounting system is a strict one and a shortage of fluid on any one day remains in arrears until it is replaced. Small deficiencies each day are cumulative and the sudden development of a complex fluid problem can usually trace its beginning to deficits occurring several days previously.

Reduced to its simplest terms, the major depletions can be prevented by daily determining the amount of fluid and electrolytes lost by all routes—and then replacing them. The overall view of losses of fluids and electrolytes can be grouped into three general categories, and these must be continually borne in mind in the care of any sick individual.

1. Daily obligatory losses.
2. Additional routes of loss.
3. Effect of kidney function and stress.

OBLIGATORY LOSSES AND GAINS OF FLUID

If an individual were to stop all fluid intake there would continue to be a daily loss of 1,500 cc. for excretory purposes. This may be called the obligatory fluid loss. It is the sum of water lost by evaporation from the skin and the moisture of respiration (900 cc.), and the smallest amount of urine required to excrete the waste of a day's metabolism (600 cc.). This amount of fluid, 1,500 cc., is the minimum quantity which an adult requires to maintain himself in balance. Should the quantity of loss be increased by additional losses from other sources or if his kidneys are not concentrating at peak efficiency, then this amount would not be sufficient for daily requirements.

If the patient is able to eat he will gain a volume of water which is equal to the weight of the food, since for practical calculation food may be recorded as water. Thus, 1,000 Gm. of solids is included as 1,000 cc. of water. A patient who is eating a normal diet, therefore, will require a minimum of 500 cc. of fluid to replace his obligatory fluid losses. If he is taking nothing orally, then the full 1,500 cc. of fluid must be given parenterally. Besides the actual water content of food, a small amount of extra water is gained as the fats, proteins and carbohydrates are oxidized and new water molecules are formed. This quantity is small (100 to 200 cc.) and is about equal to the amount of fluid lost in normal feces. Therefore, in the absence of diarrhea this gain and loss cancel out and may be ignored. In a similar manner, the fasting individual gains a small amount of water released with protoplasmic breakdown and from metabolism of the endogenous proteins and fats, but this too may be ignored in clinical computation.

Fluid of Perspiration and Urine

The losses of fluid from the body, which actually occur, usually are more than the minimal obligatory losses. Fever, work, hot weather and shocklike states may increase greatly the amount of evaporative loss both from rapid respiration and from the formation of visible sweat. Several liters per day may be lost in this manner. If visible perspiration is evident during the course of a day one may add 1,000 cc. or more to the loss column. It is estimated that a single change of bed clothes represents at least a liter of water lost.

The actual output of urine is considerably more than the minimum of 600 cc. and usually averages between 1,000 to 1,500 cc. daily. The volume of urine will depend on the amount of water ingested, the amount of waste to be excreted and the

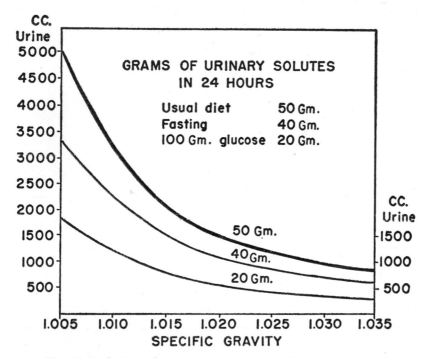

Fig. 9. Relation of urine volume to specific gravity at given urinary solute loads. The solute load of the urine is the metabolic waste which is composed largely of urea and electrolytes. With good concentrating ability, 50 Gm. of solutes can be excreted in 800 cc. of urine. At a specific gravity of only 1.010, however, this same solute load requires about 3,500 cc. A fasting individual has a 40 Gm. solute load, the result of endogenous protein preakdown. Administration of 100 Gm. of glucose reduces this to 20 Gm. by its protein-sparing effect. If the maximum concentrating ability of the kidney is known, the necessary volume of urine can be determined for the known solute load. (After Gamble)

ability of the kidneys to concentrate the urine (Fig. 9). The metabolic wastes (solutes) which are dissolved in the urine are largely nitrogenous end products (urea) and electrolytes, with the total quantity of these resulting from the average diet being about 40 to 50 Gm. If the amount of water available for excretion is large, these 50 Gm. are diluted in a large volume of urine and the specific gravity of the urine is low (below 1.010). If the amount of fluid available is small, however, the 50 Gm. of solutes may be excreted in as little as 600 cc. of concentrated urine at a specific gravity of 1.035 or more. Kidneys which are unable to concentrate will need larger amounts of fluid to excrete the same amount of solute; this must be accomplished by consuming more water. Failing in this, and in order to supply the needed volume of urine, fluid will be drawn from the tissues, thus eventually leading to dehydration. However, if the fluid is not available from the body, because of already existing dehydration, the metabolic wastes can not be excreted, and they become manifest as a rising blood urea nitrogen or NPN. The fact that edema is present does not alter this requirement for extra fluid where the concentrating power of the kidney is impaired, and additional water must be given regardless of the presence of edema. The ability of the kidney to concentrate may be impaired, either permanently or temporarily, in chronic nephritis, arteriosclerotic kidneys, diabetes insipidus, severe emotional disturbances, in newborns and in the recovery phase of lower nephron nephrosis. Therefore, the daily water requirement will be increased in these individuals.

The fact that the patient is not eating does not appreciably change water requirements for excretion of metabolites. In the fasting state the solute load is about 40 Gm. a day and represents the end products of tissue protein breakdown and excess ketone formation. If 100 Gm. of glucose are supplied to the fasting patient daily, the protein-sparing effect of this caloric addition reduces the solute load to 20 Gm. Figure 9 shows the fluid requirement for excreting this amount of solute. As a corollary to this, excessive loss of fluid leading to dehydration may occur as a result of increased solute loads. For example, in fever, severe muscular exertion and in thyrotoxicosis the increased metabolic turnover requires a greater urine output to handle the increased amount of metabolites. Uncontrolled diabetes causes polyuria by increasing the solute load of glucose.

Although inadequate fluid intake results in a small volume of urine, conversely, the presence of a small urine volume does not necessarily indicate a small intake of fluid. Diversion of fluid into other channels as in edema or ascites formation or loss of fluid by other routes, such as in profuse perspiration or diarrhea will leave less fluid available for urine formation. In effect, the kidneys get the fluid which is left over after all other fluid losses have been met.

In summary, then, the amount of fluid to replace obligatory loss is adequate only if there is no visible perspiration and if the kidneys are functioning at top concentrating capacity. In order to insure adequate urine output and to decrease the work of the kidney, an additional amount of fluid over that necessary to replace obligatory loss should be allowed. If impairment of concentrating ability exists, this can be compensated by giving an extra liter of fluid daily.

LOSSES WITHIN THE BODY

The accumulation of dependent edema fluid and ascites, although these remain within the body, involves the loss of this fluid for ordinary bodily functions (such as urine excretion and sweating). These accumulations may grow at the expense of the extracellular fluid. Crushing injuries, severe burns, peritonitis and massive thrombophlebitis also produce losses of fluid as localized edema accumulates at the site of the injury. In intestinal obstruction the fluid accumulation in the distended loops of the bowel are true losses as far as fluid balance is concerned and will lead to rapid dehydration. An additional intake must be allowed for replacement of the fluid lost in these dislocations.

SODIUM INTAKE AND OUTPUT

The important role of sodium in maintaining blood volume and regulation of fluid osmolarity has been discussed and, as one might suspect from this, the total body sodium must be carefully preserved. The average diet contains about 10 Gm. of salt, the greatest part of which is excreted in the urine. If the intake of food and salt stops, the urinary output of sodium rapidly decreases and in 4 to 5 days becomes negligible. Since the amount of sodium lost in invisible perspiration and feces is very small, a normal individual may get along for considerable periods of time with a low salt intake *if* there are no other routes of loss. The use of mercurial diuretics interferes with the ability of the kidney to conserve sodium so that cessation of intake in individuals receiving diuretics will lead to rapid depletion. In Addison's disease and in "salt-losing nephritis" there is likewise an inability to retain sodium, so that even with normal intake salt depletion will occur.

Visible sweat is a hypotonic solution which averages about 50 mEq. of sodium per liter. In hot weather the loss of several liters daily may lead to appreciable salt deficits in normal individuals, and especially so in patients on salt-restricted diets or those receiving diuretics. Acclimatization to heat over long periods of time will reduce the sodium content of sweat to about 5 mEq./L., which is the amount contained in invisible perspiration. This is not apt to occur in the period of a few summer months, however.

POTASSIUM GAIN AND LOSS

Potassium is present in large quantities in many foods, with the average diet supplying 60 to 100 mEq. daily. The ability of the kidneys to save potassium is much less efficient than for sodium and even with negligible potassium intake, a urinary loss of at least 30 mEq. occurs daily. At this rate large deficits of potassium may occur in relatively few days if potassium intake is inadequate. In addition, if there is potassium loss from other sources such as occurs in diarrhea or from cellular dehydration, severe depletions may quickly occur. Potassium loss in sweat is ordinarily variable and small, but may be as much as 75 mEq./L. in visible perspiration. Mercurial diuretics may materially increase the excretion of potassium along with sodium, and when sodium deficiency exists, even larger quantities of potassium may be lost in lieu of sodium. The amount excreted in this manner is unpredictable but very large deficits have been reported. Other diuretics which cause cation loss likewise may cause potassium depletion. The use of cation exchange resins, which prevent absorption of this electrolyte from the intestine, may have a similar effect.

Important information may be gained by measuring the amount of potassium excreted in the urine as compared to nitrogen. Normally, a fairly constant ratio of 2.9 mEq. of potassium to 1 Gm. of nitrogen (K/N = 2.9) is found. This indicates a uniform cell protein breakdown. Where cellular dehydration is occurring at a rate in excess of protein breakdown the additional K^+ present in cell fluid is also lost so that the K/N excretion ratio becomes greater than 2.9.

INTESTINAL LOSSES

The output of fluid and electrolytes by the normal channels of renal and evaporative loss are strictly controlled by the body, thus preventing excessive loss of these substances. The abnormal loss which occurs from the intestinal tract, however, is without control or regard to the needs of the individual and may rapidly lead to severe imbalances. The amount of fluid lost by vomiting or diarrhea may approach 15 to 20 L. or more in severely ill patients. The obvious benefit to be gained in careful measurement of the quantity lost should be evident. If measurement is not possible, careful estimates should be made. Intestinal fluid lost by suction and indwelling tubes can and should be accurately measured.

Two types of disturbances may result from loss of large amounts of intestinal fluids. The first relates to changes in osmolarity of blood serum and is caused by the difference in concentration of sodium in the intestinal fluids as compared to blood (Table 2). In gastric juice especially, but also in the fluids obtained through the Miller-Abbott tube, the sodium concentration is lower than that of blood (hypotonic) so that for every liter of fluid lost a greater proportion of water is lost to sodium. Therefore, the resulting effect on blood osmolarity is a water depletion with elevation of sodium concentration,

MEANS OF FLUID LOSS	mEq./Liter		
	Na	*K*	*Cl*
Gastric	60	9	84
Miller-Abbott Tube	111	5	104
Ileostomy			
Recent	129	11	116
Adapted	46	3	21
Bile	148	5	100
Pancreatic	141	5	76
Diarrhea	150-350	15-70	—

TABLE 2. Average electrolyte composition of intestinal fluid (After Lockwood and Randall, and Moore). The range of values from which these figures were obtained is exceedingly broad and the average figures can therefore serve only as rough guides. Clinically, there is usually an admixture of secretions so that gastric juice can be replaced by hypotonic salt solutions, but lower intestinal secretions require isotonic salt solutions. In loss of gastric and pancreatic juice, alkalosis or acidosis results, respectively, because of the disproportion of sodium and chloride.

although total body sodium is lessened. In the bile and pancreatic juices, which make up a large part of diarrhea fluid, the sodium concentration is equal to or greater than that of blood (isotonic or hypertonic). The effect on extracellular fluid, therefore, is to decrease volume with no change in osmolarity, or, in diarrhea, to cause salt depletion with a lower sodium concentration.

The second type of disturbance resulting from loss of large amounts of intestinal fluid has to do with alteration of electrolyte equilibrium affecting acid-base balance. In gastric juice the amount of chloride is much greater than sodium as compared to the reverse state in blood. Therefore, vomiting or gastric tube suction will lead to large chloride deficits with resulting alkalosis. However, pancreatic juice has a preponderance of sodium to chloride, with considerable bicarbonate as well, so that diarrhea leads to base deficits with resulting acidosis.

Since electrolyte concentration of the various intestinal juices is extremely variable within wide limits and there is apt to be considerable admixture of different secretions, chemical determination is the only method of accurately establishing the true losses. If chemical methods are not available a rough approximation should be attempted from the table of average compositions (Table 2).

The potassium concentration in intestinal fluids is usually somewhat higher than the concentration in blood serum, but, with vomiting and diarrhea, concentrations up to 80 mEq./L. may be lost. The loss of this electrolyte in intestinal fluids is the reason for the large deficits of potassium which have been reported in infantile and adult diarrhea.

STRESS REACTIONS

The urinary excretion of sodium and potassium are altered markedly by trauma or stress, whether this be a cholecystectomy, surgical anesthesia, coronary occlusion or exposure to cold. These effects must be considered in planning the therapy of such patients. It has been shown by Moore that the immediate response to any severe traumatizing episode is really the end result of several factors, namely, tissue damage, starvation, immobilization and endocrines. The electrolytes are particularly influenced by the endocrine factor as a result of the "stress reaction" (Selye). Many workers have verified the fact that in response to any stress there is a release of ACTH (adrenocorticotropic hormone) from the pituitary. This hormone stimulates the adrenal cortex which in turn secretes its several types of steroids (Fig. 10). One of these, the electrolyte hormone, (desoxicorticosterone-like or mineral-corticoids) causes diminished sodium excretion both by the kidney and the sweat glands, and indirectly increases the loss of potassium. A second hormone, the "sugar hormone" (compounds E and F, cortisone or glucocorticoids), has a mineral-corticoidlike action, likewise causing sodium retention and potassium loss. This hormone also has a marked catabolic (antianabolic) effect which prevents the buildup of proteins. Thus amino acids are made available at the site of injury for tissue repair and also for conversion to glucose (hence "sugar hormone"). Elevation of the blood sugar for immediate energy requirements following stress is a measure of this protein-conversion-to-glucose (gluconeogenesis) and is not indicative of latent diabetes. It has been suggested that the salt retention and potassium loss (releasing cell water) were purposely designed to maintain the blood volume in time of stress, as well as to supply the elements for healing to the area of damage at the expense of the general body mass. This chain reaction of stress and the release of "sugar hormone" can be identified to some extent by the drop in number of circulating eosinophils in the blood. It is possible to determine the adequacy of adrenal cortical function by following the postoperative drop in eosinophil count, although the degree of drop is not a quantitative measure of response. That is, additional injury may cause additional hor-

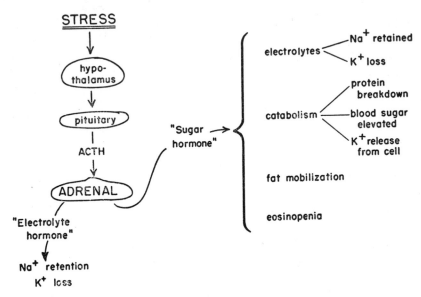

Fig. 10. Effect of stress on electrolyte excretion. In the attempt to maintain homeostasis, any traumatic episode will produce a series of endocrine effects resulting in sodium (Na^+) retention and potassium (K^+) loss. The degree and duration of the effects are roughly proportional to the severity and duration of the trauma and ordinarily last 2 to 5 days. The ability of the adrenals to respond to a trauma may be measured by the drop in total eosinophils and by their return to normal levels as the patient recovers.

mone release which can not be reflected further in a drop in eosinophils which are already low.

The duration of the sodium retention and potassium loss will depend to a great extent on the severity of the trauma. Ordinarily the adrenal response will last for about 2 to 5 days at which time the eosinophil count is back to normal. The immediate post-traumatic period is followed by a repair period in which there is a sodium diuresis and potassium retention. The amount of potassium retention during the postoperative convalescence indicates that there has been intracellular potassium loss over that which might be expected as a result of protein breakdown, and, is indicative therefore, of cell water loss.

If adrenal function is inadequate the sodium retention will not occur and salt depletion will result if sodium is withheld. The persistent output of over 40 mEq./L. of sodium in the urine in the presence of a low serum sodium is diagnostic of adrenal cortical insufficiency. Failure of circulating eosinophils to drop postoperatively will likewise identify this condition.

CHAPTER FOUR

Prevention of Imbalance in the Postoperative Patient

In balancing the income and outgo one must be continually aware of the avenues of gain and loss. In summary form these are:

AVENUES OF GAIN	AVENUES OF LOSS	
	Normal	*Abnormal*
1. Mouth	1. Urine, affected by	3. Intestinal losses
Food (weight)	Renal function	Vomiting,
Water	Stress	intubation
2. Parenteral solution	2. Evaporation	Diarrhea
	Perspiration	Fistula
	Respiration	4. Internal fluid shifts
		Edema, ascites,
		peritonitis
		Crushes, severe
		trauma
		Burns
		5. Surgical or trau-
		matic loss
		Blood loss
		Evaporation
		(wound)

The clinical importance of stress on sodium and potassium excretion in postoperative electrolyte management is demonstrated in two simple surgical cases. One patient received, postoperatively, 2,500 cc. of glucose in water daily and the other was given the same volume of fluid, but 1,500 cc. of isotonic saline was included. In the first case (Fig. 11) the sodium excretion dropped promptly following surgery as the body defenses were geared to salt conservation, and in the period of 4 days after surgery there was a minimal deficit of sodium in the body. Potassium excretion was increased over the preoperative rate. A slight drop in the hematocrit was evident, which usually occurs postoperatively as a result of expansion of the blood volume (the effect of salt retention). In the second case (Fig. 12), the excretion of sodium lagged far behind the amount of sodium which was administered and resulted in a considerable excess of retained sodium in the 4-day postoperative period. This was reflected in the very appreciable drop in hematocrit resulting from dilution of the blood with the added fluids. Potassium excretion again showed the increased daily loss of about 60 mEq.

While such an excess of salt could well be handled by the individual under ordinary circumstances, this may not hold true in many other conditions. The patient with myocardial damage might easily be pushed into acute pulmonary edema by this degree of blood volume expansion. The traumatic edema which occurs at the site of intestinal anastomoses, if augmented by salt-produced edema, might result in closure of the stoma with an unwarranted surgical failure. Postoperative salt retention is also a hazard in neurosurgery in the production of excessive brain edema. Balance studies have shown that similar electrolyte changes occur following thoracic surgery. Potassium deficits may be less marked here, however, since loss of intestinal secretion is not a factor. With poor respiratory reserve and with postoperative anoxia in these patients, even minimal edema brought on by salt administration postoperatively may produce serious pulmonary edema.

Intake and output are so automatically adjusted in the normal individual that generally there is a tendency to ignore

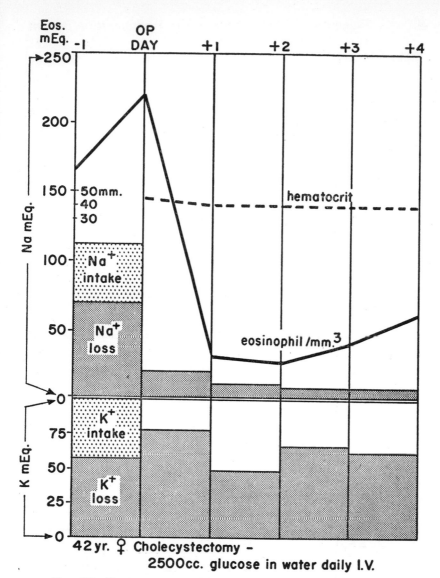

FIG. 11. Postoperative electrolyte loss in urine. Water replacement. The adrenal response in this patient is evident from the posttraumatic drop in eosinophil count which persisted for the 4-day study. The postoperative retention of sodium (Na+) prevents excessive loss of this ion, so that blood volume is maintained in time of stress. The drop in hematocrit indicates blood volume expansion which is the result of the sodium retention. Potassium (K+) excretion increases following surgery and is the result of cell protein breakdown and loss of intracellular water.

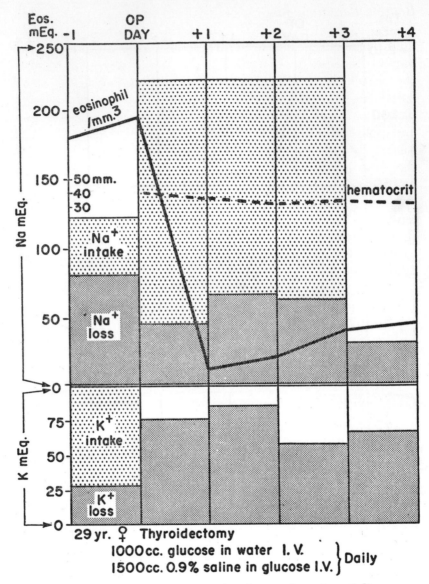

FIG. 12. Postoperative electrolyte loss in the urine. Saline replacement. The adrenal response is shown by the eosinophil count drop. The retention of sodium (Na+) is augmented by the intravenous saline solutions so that by the end of the third postoperative day a great excess of sodium has accumulated in the body. The marked drop in hematocrit is the result of blood dilution with the added saline. Potassium (K+) excretion is augmented by intravenous salt administration which diureses the potassium from the cells.

fluid balance until it is brought forcibly to our attention as the patient becomes more critically ill. If the physician applies the principles of normal intake and output and keeps these equal there is ordinarily little difficulty in keeping the average patient in good fluid balance. The physiologic salt retention and potassium loss after surgery (or other trauma) is well tolerated by most patients for a period of several days even if these are not corrected in the therapy. However, if attention has not been given to proper maintenance in the early postoperative care, unforeseen prolongation of the need for parenteral feedings (postoperative infection, dehiscence or further surgery) may precipitate an embarrassing severe water or electrolyte depletion, which has been gradually developing over several days.

ROUTINE REQUIREMENTS

Based upon the physiologic principles which have been presented one can arrive at a rational program of routine treatment for the uncomplicated surgical (or medical) patient who requires parenteral fluid. It should be stressed that although many of these do well in spite of improper fluid balance, complications occurring 3 to 4 days postoperatively may become much more hazardous if fluid imbalance has been permitted to develop. Once a patient begins to eat adequately, existing imbalances are generally spontaneously repaired providing circulation and kidney function are normal. The following are considered to be the essentials for proper maintenance therapy.

FLUIDS

The minimum fluid intake should be 2,500 cc. daily.

This will cover the obligatory loss of fluids by invisible perspiration and moisture of respiration and will supply enough water to permit the renal excretion of about 1,500 cc. of urine. This is sufficient fluid to excrete the average amount of urinary wastes even with some impairment of the kidney's ability to concentrate. If the renal disease is severe with a fixed specific gravity at 1.010, an additional 500 cc. of water should be allowed. To replace evaporative loss from the surgical field an additional 1,000 cc. is given on the day of surgery, ordinarily during the course of the operation.

In addition, any deficit of fluid carried over from the previous day must be given, along with any special anticipated losses for the current 24-hour period. Anticipated losses might be fluid loss from a draining fistula, intestinal intubation, excessive perspiration, etc. Excess water given on previous days cannot be deducted, since it will have been excreted as urine at the time given. It is well to pay attention to the patient's desires as far as fluid is concerned. A complaint of thirst more than likely means that he needs water. The patient does not usually confuse a dry mouth with actual thirst.

Sodium

No salt solution is given for from 2 to 5 days.

For several days postoperatively, or following any traumatic episode such as coronary occlusion, severe fracture, etc., no sodium need be given because of physiologic sodium retention under these circumstances. Of course, this does not obviate the need for replacing any sodium which may be lost in intestinal secretions. In the absence of accurate measurement of sodium loss from intestinal sources, a rough approximation may be attempted by giving volume for volume of hypotonic saline (4.5 Gm./L.) for gastric loss, or isotonic saline (9 Gm./L.) for lower intestinal loss. In the immediate postoperative period there is more danger from too much, rather than from too little sodium.

If parenteral feeding is still necessary following the post-traumatic period of sodium retention, 500 cc. of normal saline (4.5 Gm. of NaCl) will more than adequately cover the usual daily loss, and, here again, extra loss from the intestine must also be added. Other available solutions which are more physiologic will be discussed in a later chapter (Chap. 9). To avoid the danger of overhydration from too much saline, it is best not to anticipate sodium loss, but rather to replace the losses of the previous day.

POTASSIUM

Give 40 mEq. daily as long as parenteral feeding is necessary.

It is important to make certain of an adequate urine output before administering potassium. For this reason it should be withheld in the immediate post-traumatic period until an adequate urine flow has been verified (Chap. 7). The daily requirement may be given in the intravenous fluids, 20 mEq. in each liter (as potassium chloride or potassium phosphate), although 40 mEq./L. is quite safe given at 90 drops per minute.

Intestinal secretions may contain considerable amounts of potassium and will need replacement, especially in severe diarrheas. In the absence of actual measurement of potassium loss, an additional 20 to 40 mEq. may be given for each liter of secretion lost. If urine volume is adequate any excess of potassium which may have been given will be excreted. When oral feedings are taken it is no longer necessary to give potassium since most diets contain large amounts of this element. Prophylaxis of potassium depletion should begin when the intestinal tube suction and intravenous fluids are administered.

GLUCOSE

At least 100 Gm. daily in intravenous solution is needed.

This amount of glucose (1 L. of 5 per cent glucose has 50 Gm.) minimizes protein breakdown and resulting fluid and potassium loss. This is also of advantage in anurias and in impending uremias since it reduces nitrogenous waste by its protein-sparing effect. The movement of potassium into the cell does not occur in the absence of adequate amounts of glucose and insulin.

BLOOD

Blood transfusion replaces blood volume, not fluid needs.

When blood is given for either replacement of blood loss or other reasons it is not to be considered part of the daily fluid intake. Since it is fully constituted as to cells, protein and electrolytes, it serves to make up blood volume but does not supply free water for urinary or sweat requirement, nor does it supply extra salt or other electrolytes.

INTESTINAL SUCTION

Use hypotonic saline for irrigation.

Aggravation of electrolyte loss may occur in patients with intestinal intubation by frequent irrigation of the tube. Tap water or electrolyte-free solutions used for irrigation, dilute the intestinal secretions and make them hypotonic. This acts as a stimulus for more secretion of electrolytes by the intestinal mucosa and the tap water is then sucked out with an additional load of electrolytes. The same fault occurs when patients are permitted to drink copiously of water while such tubes are functioning. The author recalls a patient who was permitted to drink 21 L. (!) of water which promptly ran out of the tube, leaving the patient with a profound alkalosis from which he never recovered. The rule then is not to permit more than occasional sips of water while suction tubes are operating.

PREVENTION OF IMBALANCE IN COMPLICATED SURGICAL CASES

In postoperative patients requiring intestinal intubation or in those with indwelling drainage tubes or fistulae, the problem of maintaining electrolyte balance becomes more complex. In the absence of chemical determinations one can at least attempt approximations of the electrolyte loss from the known average concentrations (Table 2) of intestinal juices. Somewhat better estimates may be obtained by measuring the chloride output in urine and intestinal secretions by the simple Fantus chloride test. This is of limited value since, as will be shown, the output of chloride only roughly parallels the sodium excretion in urine and is at considerable variance with sodium in intestinal fluids. A system of clinical fluid and electrolyte balance has been described by Scribner utilizing a modification of the chloride excretion as the basis for replacement of lost electrolytes. The method works best in the hands of those well-versed in the physiology of abnormal electrolyte structure. Recently, Talbott and King have described a simple bedside method of analysis which gives a roughly quantitative determination of sodium. Since the determination is based on precipitation of sodium as the zinc uranyl acetate, a turbid or cloudy test solution will interfere with the test. This can be corrected by filtering the urine, but the value of the test on intestinal fluids is questionable.

With the more universal availability of the flame photometer the problem of determination of electrolytes in body fluids has been much simplified, so that the determination of potassium and sodium can now be performed in a matter of minutes. It is the author's belief that where major surgery is being routinely performed, the determination of electrolytes by flame photometry is as important to the management of many of these patients as is the blood sugar in the diabetic in acidosis. The author has described a clinical fluid and electrolyte service based on the actual determination of sodium and potassium lost in urine and intestinal fluids. The value of this method is its accuracy in measuring losses as compared to the other systems and the simplicity of performance. For the details in the several methods of management the reader is referred to the original descriptions.

CHAPTER FIVE

Water Depletion

The confusion that still exists in the diagnosis of the major fluid imbalances is evident when one frequently witnesses the administration of antibiotics for the fever of dehydration, the use of the Miller-Abbott tube for the distention of potassium depletion and the diagnosis of cerebrovascular accident or heart failure for the shocklike state of salt depletion. It is important to recognize the fact that a fluid or electrolyte imbalance may be present regardless of the nature of the original illness, since in any sick individual the intake of food and water is apt to be interrupted. One needs to see only once the hourly dramatic improvement of an almost moribund patient to be convinced of the importance of recognizing these deficiencies and their proper correction.

A good history and physical examination will give more information in determining the existing state of fluid balance than most laboratory tests which are performed. With a complete tabulation of what the patient has been eating and drinking over the previous several days, and with the general appearance and examination of the individual one can identify

the nature of the deficit which has already developed. This
will give the basis for *what* the patient needs therapeutically,
and then it remains only to decide *how much*. The writer has
found Marriott's classification of the degree of depletion to be
simple and accurate enough for most clinical purposes. From
the symptoms and examination one can estimate the amount
of deficit and thus have a rational basis for approximating replacement solutions. Laboratory tests are a help and give the
fine adjustment to accurate diagnosis, but are not absolutely
necessary for proper therapy.

CAUSES

The picture of water depletion is found as the result of water
loss without adequate replacement or, when both water and
salt are being lost, the water wastage occurring in excess of the
salt. In elderly people and in patients with clouded sensorium,
confused states and psychoses, there is frequently neglect of
fluid intake when left to their own efforts. In patients with
debilitating illnesses, such as protracted infections, carcinoma,
chronic painful diseases, sore throats and in status asthmaticus
there is interference with the normal desires for food and drink.
Dehydration develops in all of these because fluid is not being
taken in spite of the fact that obligatory losses are still going on.

Besides the above group one finds water depletion in patients who are losing hypotonic fluid from the body so that
water loss is therefore exceeding the rate of salt loss. This
occurs in the severe sweating of fever or in hot weather, and
with the gastric juice loss of vomiting or gastric suction. Obligatory fluid loss in addition to this puts the deficit of water
far ahead of the sodium want. Improper postoperative fluid
replacement, by ignoring evaporative losses, is one of the commonest causes of water depletion seen in hospital patients.

FLUID SHIFTS

The physiologic changes resulting from the imbalance, (Fig.
13), are similar to the changes described in the Darrow and
Yannet experiments (Chap. 2). As fluid is lost from the extracellular space, the plasma sodium concentration is increased,

producing what Darrow speaks of as "hypertonic dehydration."
The fluid loss leads to a drop in blood volume which, by way
of adrenal action, promotes a more marked sodium retention
(dehydration reaction). This salt conservation serves a double
purpose in that less water is being wasted in excreting the
sodium, and as the plasma osmolarity increases with the retained sodium, water is drawn from the cells, thereby depleting
them but augmenting the lessened blood volume. In later
stages, as the blood volume continues to diminish, the plasma
proteins become more concentrated and cause a shift of fluid
into the blood vessels from the relatively protein-free interstitial compartment. This mechanism is also important in maintaining the blood volume (Fig. 8). In the early dehydration
occurring in the first two days the fluid which is lost is derived
in equal quantities from both major fluid compartments, but in
chronic dehydration the cellular loss becomes predominant.
The important ultimate effect, therefore, is a *more or less pro-*

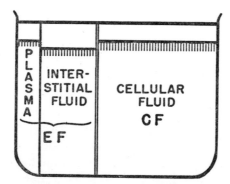

Fig. 13. Body fluid compartments
in water depletion. The EF becomes hypertonic and the resulting
osmotic pressure causes a withdrawal of fluid from the CF. The
fluid loss in water depletion is,
therefore, proportionate from all
compartments. Loss of cell fluid involves the substances dissolved in it
and, thus, potassium, magnesium
and some protein are lost as well.

portionate loss of fluid from both major fluid compartments;
cellular fluid as well as extracellular fluid being lost in water
depletion. The substances dissolved or suspended in the cell
fluid (potassium, magnesium, phosphates and, to a less extent,
protein) are lost with the cellular water. During starvation,
but without water deprivation, the loss of cell protoplasm will
be accompanied by the amount of fluid in which the protein
is suspended. There will be no dehydration and no hypertonicity of body fluids. In primary water depletion, however,
the loss of fluid is excessive and, although accompanied by
some protoplasmic breakdown, the amount of protein lost is
small in comparison to the fluid volume loss.

BLOOD AND URINE PICTURE

Even though there is an actual decrease in the total amount
of sodium remaining in the body, the serum sodium level will
be elevated since water has been lost in excess of sodium. An
elevated serum sodium *always* means water depletion, but the
degree of elevation is only roughly proportional to the degree
of dehydration, since one does not know how much more
water has been lost than salt. One possible exception is the
hypernatremia in diseases involving the hypothalamus or
frontal lobes of the brain. The administration of extra water
here does not lower the sodium concentration. If the urinary
excretion of potassium has not kept pace with the large potassium losses from within the cells, the serum potassium will be
elevated, even though a large potassium deficit exists. Similar
changes occur with magnesium. The hematocrit and plasma
proteins are elevated late as a result of hemoconcentration.
Blood volume is partially maintained early at the expense
of the interstitial fluid because of the protein effect. When
low grade dehydration has been present for longer periods
of time, the homeostatic mechanisms of the body will adjust
the elevated protein and blood cell concentration. The protein level drops to its normal range and the excess red cells
are destroyed, so that a normal blood count results. Sudden
re-expansion of blood volume by intravenous fluids at this
time, will result in a hypoproteinemia and an anemia by its
diluting effect.

In dehydration the urine soon becomes concentrated with a high specific gravity and of small volume, depending on the ability of the kidneys to concentrate. If the solute load is high, as, for example, in the glycosuria of diabetes, the volume may still be large in spite of severe dehydration. An adequate urine volume, therefore, does not exclude the diagnosis of dehydration. Signs of renal injury may be present with red blood cells and casts as a manifestation of the dehydration. The excretion of sodium and chloride in the urine is normal in the early stages, but, as the blood volume drops, the urinary sodium is diminished although blood levels are elevated.

CLINICAL PICTURE

If the clinical picture can be converted into terms of the per cent of body weight lost, one then readily has available a rough guide for replacement therapy. Thus, a loss of 5 per cent of body weight in a 70 Kg. patient indicates a deficit of 3.5 L. of fluid, which in water depletion has derived from both of the major fluid compartments. As described above, only a small fraction of this weight loss is protein loss. It is of great practical value, then, to familiarize oneself with the symptoms in mild, marked and severe dehydration (after Marriott).

Mild Dehydration (2 per cent of body weight lost).

The earliest indication of water depletion is thirst, which is symptomatic of relatively minute water deficits and which may remain the only symptom for up to 1 to 2 L. of water deficit. Thirst is not specific for fluid loss, however, since it may be found also as a symptom of large hemorrhages and nervousness, or it may be simple habit.

Marked Dehydration (5 per cent of body weight lost).

The patient seen in the home who has been ill for 3 or 4 days prior to seeking medical help will often present this picture. The symptoms are marked thirst with dry mucous membranes, so that speaking is difficult without first moistening the mouth. The patient looks weak and ill, and in spite of this is restless. The loss of weight is proportional to the amount of fluid deficit. There is tachycardia as the blood volume begins to drop and low grade elevation of temperature is common. The urine is small in volume and highly concentrated (specific gravity over 1.035) if the kidneys are competent. The practicing physician will recognize this clinical picture as one commonly seen and it is one worth remembering. It indicates a deficit of about 3 to 5 L. of fluid.

Severe Dehydration (8 per cent of body weight lost).

In addition to the symptoms already enumerated the skin becomes flushed and mental symptoms become most prominent. Marked restlessness, change of personality and, later, disorientation, delirium, mania, coma and death finally occur. With the progressive drop in blood volume, a drop in blood pressure occurs with tachycardia. The temperature becomes high terminally. The cause of death in severe dehydration is largely because of interference with the metabolic processes as the result of the intracellular dessication. These changes represent a water loss of 5 to 10 L.

REQUIREMENTS OF THERAPY

It is evident that the picture of water depletion is in reality a rather complex multiple depletion syndrome. Fluids need to be replaced to the extent of the total weight loss. Sodium has been lost from the extracellular fluid, although there is an elevated serum sodium, and if water alone is given in therapy a moderate salt depletion will be the end result. Along with the loss of cellular fluid, potassium will be excreted in the face of an elevated serum potassium, and replacement therapy with saline solution alone will not only make the potassium deficit manifest by diluting the blood serum, but will also aggravate the deficiency by diuresing more potassium as the sodium replaces it in the cell (Chap. 8).

In chronic dehydration, the loss of protein and red cells will lead to hypoproteinemia and anemia when fluids are restored, unless whole blood is also given. Loss of cellular fluid has also contributed to protoplasmic breakdown with some protein deficits, and this probably accounts for a fraction of the weight loss.

CHAPTER SIX

Salt Depletion

In salt depletion, an accurate history of the onset of the illness, with an inquiry into the food and fluid ingested over the several previous days, will give a fairly adequate impression of the character and degree of the imbalance. As in water depletion, a good approximation of the magnitude of the deficit can be obtained from the symptoms and physical findings. One should not depend on laboratory procedures alone. A low serum sodium is not necessarily indicative of salt depletion. In the chapters on edema and cardiac disease are discussed several instances of low serum sodium which are not associated with a total salt deficit in the body generally. In the present discussion those instances where the deficits of sodium have developed in comparatively short periods of time are being specifically referred to.

CAUSES

Since there is no obligatory loss of salt as there is for fluid and since loss of hypertonic fluids from the body is unusual, the development of salt depletion is less often a result of omission and not infrequently one of commission, by the doctor especially. It occurs where the rate of salt loss exceeds water loss, as in severe diarrhea, or where both salt and water are being lost, but only water is being adequately replaced. Excessive perspiring during hot weather and fever coupled with copious water-drinking, is a cause which is frequently seen. With vomiting or diarrhea, patients are often instructed to force fluids, such as tea, carbonated drinks or fruit juices (with low salt content) where boullion or soups would be more physiologic. The recent popularity of low salt diets for cardiacs, nephritics and hypertensives, along with potent diuretics and sodium-removing exchange resins has accounted for the increased incidence of the syndrome (which is doctor induced). Patients receiving just the bare minimum of salt daily are especially susceptible to any added sodium loss such as occurs during the hot summer months or during a bout with diarrhea.

In hospital patients excessive salt loss may result from irrigation of intestinal suction tubes with tap water, a procedure which stimulates more electrolyte secretion and removal. Permitting the drinking of water or tea while suction tubes function produces the same result. The author has seen several cardiac patients in whom too rigid salt restriction postoperatively, for fear of precipitating decompensation as a result of the sodium retention of stress, led to severe salt depletions. Hypodermoclyses with 5 per cent glucose solution or other mixtures containing no salt produce a transfer of salt from the interstitial tissues into the pool of administered solution. Large losses of body sodium may be produced temporarily in this manner, and in an already salt depleted patient the added loss has precipitated death.

Inability of the kidneys to reabsorb sodium in the distal tubules, as in salt-losing nephritis, has been described. Addison's disease is in large part a low salt syndrome for the same reason, and is due to insufficient electrolyte-hormone secretion from the adrenal cortex. An unusual loss of sodium in the sweat of children with pancreatic fibrocystic disease has been described which is unrelated to either pulmonary or adrenal pathology. In these patients, as well as in some members of their family without pancreatic disease, the abnormality seems to be in the sweat gland itself.

FLUID SHIFTS

The excessive loss of salt as compared to water loss produces a lowered sodium concentration and the plasma therefore becomes hypotonic ("hypotonic dehydration" of Darrow) (Fig. 14). The lowered osmolarity, by its action on the supra-optic nuclei in the hypothalamus, inhibits the release of anti-diuretic hormone from the pituitary and water loss through the kidney is increased. This helps to return the osmolarity to normal, but diminishes blood volume as a result. The hypotonicity of the extracellular fluid causes a shift of fluid from this compartment into the cells, again diminishing the plasma

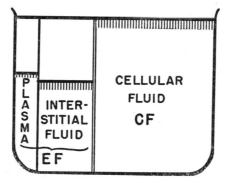

Fig. 14. Body fluid compartments and salt depletion. The EF becomes hypotonic and the osmotic pressure, therefore, causes a shift of fluid into the CF at the expense of the EF The water loss is almost entirely from the extracellular compartment. Serum protein concentration increases the tonicity of the plasma and helps replenish blood volume as fluid is drawn from the interstitial compartment. Cell fluid may be lost, also, if starvation is a factor in the development of the picture.

volume. The low blood volume results in increased sodium reabsorption by the kidney tubules (dehydration reaction) but sodium may continue to be lost by other routes (intestine). As the blood becomes more concentrated from fluid loss, the only mechanism tending to increase blood volume is the elevated plasma proteins' osmotic effect of drawing in fluid from the interstitial tissue. It has been shown that by some mechanism, not yet understood, the drop in blood volume does eventually halt the loss of fluid through the kidneys regardless of serum hypotonicity. The final picture is one of marked loss of extracellular fluid and, with this, diminished blood volume. Little if any losses occur from the cellular fluid compartment unless concomitant starvation causes protoplasmic breakdown. Where large potassium losses have occurred due to inadequate intake, the movement of sodium into the cell may aggravate the existing salt depletion. It should be noted that in the transfer of fluid from the extracellular to the cellular compartment there is no corresponding weight loss to indicate the degree of water deficit in the extracellular compartment.

BLOOD AND URINE PICTURE

The serum sodium level is low (less than 135 mEq./L.), but because of the accompanying water loss from the extracellular fluid the concentration does not give a true index of the total sodium loss. Re-expansion of the blood volume by water alone would drop the sodium level even further. The marked water loss results in hemoconcentration and all blood elements are concentrated so that blood count, hematocrit and proteins are elevated. The low blood volume and increased viscosity result in a diminished renal blood flow and the NPN or BUN become elevated. As will be shown in the chapter on acid-base balance (Chap. 8), the blood level of bicarbonate plus chloride or of chloride alone, is not a measure of sodium depletion since the uremia and alterations in the pH may change the concentration of these electrolytes without regard to the sodium level. The urine volume in these patients is unaffected early, but later becomes scant and the sodium and chlorides are absent.

The delayed diuresis after a dose of water seen in these individuals is typical also of Addison's disease and is an attempt to maintain blood volume even though the serum sodium concentration is low. Evidence of renal damage may appear with red cells, albumin and casts.

CLINICAL PICTURE

Here again an estimate of the quantitative salt deficit can be made from the clinical picture as described by Marriott. The essential symptoms and findings are those related to the drop in blood volume leading to the picture of medical shock.

Mild Salt Depletion (20 Gm. of salt deficit).

The early symptoms of salt depletion recalls one's own sensations during the course of a month in hot midsummer. Apathy, lassitude and weakness are common complaints with loss of interest in the usual activities. Dull throbbing headaches and faintness are the result of low blood volume and are often associated with loss of appetite. Thirst is ordinarily not present. With the sudden drinking of water or after sudden exertion muscle cramps may occur. These are characteristic of the stoker's cramps of salt deficiency.

Marked Salt Depletion (35 Gm. of salt deficit).

The above complaints are accentuated and profound weakness becomes the dominant symptom. Anorexia gives way to nausea and vomiting which aggravates the salt loss by a refusal to take water or food. The low blood volume begins to manifest itself in dizziness and an easily collapsible pulse, postural or orthostatic hypotension and fainting. Severe headaches become continuous and the blood pressure drops to about 100 mm. systolic. The skin is obviously dehydrated and shrunken and lack of skin turgor (pinching up the skin leaves it elevated) is due to loss of interstitial fluid. The reflexes are also diminished.

Severe Salt Depletion (50 Gm. of salt deficit).

The apathy progresses to stupor, semicoma and coma. The pulse becomes faint as the blood volume diminishes and the syncope resulting from the hypotension occurs even without postural change. The muscles are flaccid and atonic and the reflexes are absent. The urine flow is now minimal and the blood pressure is ordinarily below 90 mm. systolic. In general, the developing picture is one very similar to the addisonian crisis; that is, a picture of medical shock due to salt loss with low blood volume. This is apparently the maximum salt deficit which has been found to occur in adults.

UNUSUAL TYPES OF SALT DEPLETION

Ladell has described a type of salt depletion seen as the result of prolonged hot weather which occurs late in the summer. It usually occurs in individuals who have withstood the earlier heat without difficulty. There is a cessation of sweating, often sudden, in these people which is accompanied by the onset of frequency of urination. The main complaints are dizziness, anorexia, insomnia and dyspnea and paresthesias are common. Blood sodium levels are low but not as marked as in the usual salt depletion picture. Chloride is present in the urine in spite of low blood sodium levels. This probably represents a type of adrenal exhaustion which would best explain the picture with continued chloride loss.

A type of hyponatremia has recently been studied by Sims, et al., in which serum sodium levels of 122 to 131 mEq./L. have been found but without the clinical manifestations of true sodium depletion. These have been reported by others in patients with pulmonary tuberculosis, but it has been found also in patients exhibiting poor nutrition and in surgical patients with long standing or chronic salt depletion. There is apparently no evidence of contraction of the blood volume in these patients, and both adrenal and kidney function have not shown any abnormality. On a low salt diet the urine becomes salt free. It has been postulated that in these patients a new level of osmolarity has been set by the osmostat so that the extracellular fluid volume is maintained in spite of diminished tonicity of the blood. Administration of additional salt causes an increased excretion of sodium in the urine, but with no change in serum sodium levels. If the sodium is not excreted, edema results.

In patients who have had a major operation or suffered severe trauma, one may find what has been called a "sodium paradox." In spite of post-traumatic salt retention by the kidneys, the serum sodium level drops to as low as 125 mEq./L. Dehydration or loss of blood volume does not exist in these patients and salt administration, therefore, is not indicated. A gradual return to normal occurs as the patient recovers. Surgical patients may show acute drop in serum sodium concentrations as the result of overdilution by administration of intravenous salt-free solutions (p. 125).

REQUIREMENTS OF THERAPY

Here again it is evident that the picture of salt depletion is in reality one of multiple deficiencies. The factor of immediate concern is the drop in blood volume and the first aim of therapy is blood replacement to restore circulating volume. Sodium then must be given to establish normal osmolarity and remove fluid from the overhydrated cells, but the extent of sodium depletion is not evident from the serum sodium level because of concomitant fluid loss. Fluid also must be given, since the water diuresis in early stages leaves a water deficit. Fluid replacement dilutes the viscous blood and permits adequate urine volume for readjustment of body pH. It is important that water not be replaced before sodium, however, since further sodium dilution will aggravate the symptoms and cause further shift of fluid into the cell. Intracellular protein breakdown resulting from the associated fasting may require replacement of nitrogenous substances and potassium.

√ leur n il y a manquement 0 il n en est
quelque puis se peuvent - elle se crater il y aura donc pollution
d'être dans le sang été du NPN .

Parler dans le corps -
Lecteur et l'avez té constituent une perte de liquide ; il en est
ainsi dans le écrasement , brûlures feu treton l'obstruction
ni lutiencahe -

Une dieté moyenne contient 10 gm de sel (sodium) par an
en grande perte se crête dans l'urine -

La dacardier amenen une perte de potassim -

H.

La police est entrée en vigueur tel que mentionné dans la brochure: le 15 NOVEMBRE 1955.

Afin de permettre à un plus grand nombre d'adhérer au plan, une période d'extension d'inscription vient d'être accordée. Les membres éligibles qui soumettront leur demande d'ici le 15 FEVRIER 1956, seront acceptés indépendamment de leur état de santé, pourvu que le pourcentage d'adhésions atteigne 50% durant cette période de prolongation d'inscription.

Complétez et faites parvenir la formule de proposition insérée dans la brochure explicative, à l'administrateur du plan, M. A. - Albert Sainte-Marie, 10560, rue Francis, Montréal 12.

Je profite de l'occasion pour vous offrir mes voeux les meilleurs et les plus sincères d'une BONNE ET HEUREUSE ANNEE "1956".

Le Secrétaire-trésorier,

L.-P. Laporte, M.D.

Fédération des Sociétés Médicales

de la Province de Québec

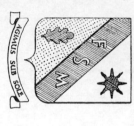

AGIMUS SUB SOLE

SIÈGE SOCIAL
ÉDIFICE DU
COLLÈGE DES MÉDECINS
1896, RUE DORCHESTER O.

MONTRÉAL,

le 30 décembre, 1955.

Mon cher confrère,

Nous avons reçu de nombreuses lettres d'appré-
ciation du PLAN EXTRAORDINAIRE d'assurance-groupe -- accident
et maladie -- spécialement préparé à l'intention des membres des sociétés médicales affiliées à la Fédération des Sociétés Médicales de
la Province de Québec.

Les inscriptions à ce plan d'assurance, dont les
CONDITIONS de contrat sont vraiment EXCEPTIONNELLES et dont

Pertes de fluides gonadiennes —
Certains produits fournis —
Effet de la fonction rénale et du foie —

Évaporation 80 c.c
urine

1800 c.c { Évaporation 800 c.c
{ urine 800 c.c

Une transpiration appréciable se fera 2.0/40 th. à une perte de 1000 c.c.

Les déchets métaboliques discrets dans l'urine sont l'urée et le chlorure ?
sont le glucose numérique et de 4/0 à 50 gm — Si l'eau supérieur
en grande quantité, ces solju seront éliminés dans un plus grand volume
d'urine mais avec une fixité spécifique de 1010 — Si l'eau ingéré
en de faible quantité les solju seront éliminés dans 600 c.c d'urine
avec une densité de 1035 —
Les reins font de pouvoir concentrer éventuellement une
densité de 10 environ de 3700 qui ne excretes de 50 gm —

CHAPTER SEVEN

Mixed Depletions, Potassium Alterations and Magnesium

MIXED DEPLETIONS

It has been pointed out that both water and salt depletion are really multiple deficiencies and the need for a mixed depletion classification may not be evident at once. In water depletion the replacement of water alone in full quantity will result in a picture of mild salt depletion. In the dehydration which results from salt loss the replacement of salt alone will leave only a moderate deficit of water. In mixed depletions, however, replacement of either substance alone will result in a rather marked deficiency of the other.

In the development of mixed depletion both are lost in large quantity but the water loss exceeds that of salt. This is because most secretions of the body, are either isotonic or hypotonic, coupled with the continued obligatory loss of water. The history of onset, as in the development of salt depletion, in most instances will reveal a loss of intestinal juices, which is the main route of abnormal salt loss. As Marriott points out, vomiting from any of its numerous causes, including pregnancy, alcoholism, any gastro-intestinal pathology and brain disease may be the initial cause of this condition. Diarrhea, draining fistulas, intestinal intubation, intestinal obstruction and diabetic coma are also frequent causes. Inadequate replacement of *both* fluid and salt leads to mixed depletion. If the patient takes fluid or is given parenteral fluids but with inadequate amounts of salt, then the picture becomes one of salt depletion.

FLUID SHIFTS

The combined spillage results in a hypertonic dehydration (Fig. 15) such as occurs in water depletion, except that the concomitant loss of salt leaves the plasma less hypertonic than is found in that condition. There is, therefore, some transfer of water from the cells and the final fluid picture is one of impoverishment in all compartments as is seen in water depletion. In addition also, there occurs the marked shrinkage of extracellular and blood volume that is found in salt deple-

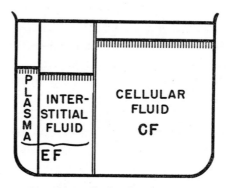

FIG. 15. Body fluid compartments in mixed depletions. The EF is hypertonic and, therefore, the cells participate in the fluid loss. The osmotic pressure of the EF is less than it might be, since large amounts of sodium have also been lost in the development of mixed depletion. All compartments lose fluid but the EF depletion is of a greater magnitude proportionately.

tion. To some extent the blood volume is protected by withdrawal of fluid from the interstitial space as the protein concentration raises the osmotic force of the plasma. The overall clinical picture resembles that of water depletion, with intracellular dehydration, but with a more rapid diminution of extracellular fluid and blood volume.

BLOOD AND URINE PICTURE

As in water depletion, the serum sodium is elevated, although not to the same degree, and again this demonstrates the inaccuracy of estimating the total body sodium deficit from the serum levels of this ion. Given the proper circumstances, a normal serum sodium level might be present with severe salt deficiency if there is coincident water lack. Blood count, protein levels and hematocrit are elevated because of hemoconcentration. The liberation of potassium from the cellular fluid and protoplasmic breakdown increases the amount of this ion in the blood, which, along with hemoconcentration and diminished urinary output incident to the low blood volume, combines to give an elevated serum potassium level. The urine shows red blood cells, albumin and casts, with the specific gravity elevated to the limit of the kidneys' ability to concentrate. The urinary chloride and sodium output is negligible.

CLINICAL PICTURE

Early in the development the symptoms are those of cellular dehydration with thirst, dry mucous membranes, weakness and flushing of the skin. As the blood volume drops, dizziness, headache and tachycardia become more prominent; a drop in blood pressure should be strong confirmatory evidence. In comparing the symptoms of mixed depletion to those of water depletion, one can, in general, follow the same classification of severity which was described in Chapter 5, to which may be added the symptoms of blood volume contraction. The site of origin of the fluid loss, for example 3,500 cc. in a marked mixed depletion, would probably partition into a somewhat greater percentage from the extracellular fluid than would be the case in water depletion. Thus, instead of one third of the total loss originating in the EF and two thirds from the CF, the loss from the two compartments would be more nearly equal.

REQUIREMENTS OF THERAPY

Again, as in primary water dehydration, fluids need to be replenished to the extent of the total weight loss, but a large amount of sodium also needs to be added. After dilution of the blood and establishment of adequate renal flow, potassium replacement must be accomplished. The loss of proteins and red cells during the development of chronic depletion warrants administration of whole blood to replace these elements. Early transfusion is of great value in restoring blood volume.

POTASSIUM ALTERATIONS

The metabolism and movement of potassium through the various body fluids is inextricably tied up with the movements of the other electrolytes and with the shifts of fluid. At this point the discussion shall bear upon the relationship of potassium to those abnormalities which have been presented already, namely, imbalances involving osmolar and volume changes. The relationship of potassium to ionic imbalances (acid-base changes) will be elaborated in the next chapter.

Certain important features of potassium physiology should be recalled: (1) the potassium concentration in the serum is low, about 5 mEq./L., (2) the concentration of potassium of the cells is high, about 150 mEq./L., (3) its concentration in intestinal secretions is ordinarily between 5 to 10 mEq./L., but with marked diarrhea may be as much as 100 mEq./L., (4) the excretion of potassium is primarily by way of the kidneys. Excesses are quickly excreted, but under conditions of deprivation there is still a continued daily loss of at least 30 mEq./L. and (5) the intracellular movement of potassium is dependent on normal cellular metabolism in the presence of oxygen and normal glucose utilization.

A restatement of the above facts reveals that, with the normal intake of about 90 mEq. daily, little alteration occurs in the blood level of potassium as it is transported to the cell or as the excess is excreted in the urine. The fact that the blood level does not reflect the large intake or the high concentration in the cell would lead one to expect that in the detection of potassium imbalances, the laboratory diagnoses, by changes in blood potassium levels, are apt to give false information. The laboratory evidence plays a subservient role to proper understanding of the clinical factors and conditions which are apt to lead to increased or decreased concentrations of potassium. In the following discussion the term hyperkalemia applies to elevation of potassium concentration in the serum and hypokalemia refers to low blood levels rather than to the amount present within the cells.

Causes of Elevation of Serum Potassium (Hyperkalemia)

A corollary to the fact that potassium is primarily excreted in the urine is the importance of an adequate urine volume to excrete the daily ingested excess. In either oliguria or anuria its concentration rises in the blood particularly if intake continues. In the absence of adrenal cortical hormones in Addison's disease, there is a tendency to potassium retention which produces no ill effects if potassium is not administered, as is done in the Cutler-Power-Wilder test of adrenal function. In the renal shutdown of "lower-nephron nephrosis" and in the anuria of acute glomerulonephritis, the hyperkalemia is not infrequently the immediate cause of death.

The serum level is also augmented in these patients by the normal metabolic processes which free potassium from cells as proteins are catabolized. Severe dehydration with release of cell water and associated cell protein destruction releases potassium into the blood, and if this dehydration is accompanied by oliguria, as it often is, the serum potassium may remain elevated until adequate water is supplied. The anhydremia which results from either water or salt depletion also concentrates the potassium and this factor is added to the dehydration effects mentioned above. In diabetic acidosis the additional factor of lack of insulin inhibits glucose utilization and thereby prevents movement of serum potassium into the cell. And lastly and most important, hyperkalemia and death may be caused by too rapid administration of potassium in intravenous solutions.

CAUSES OF POTASSIUM DEPLETION
(HYPOKALEMIA)

While high blood levels of potassium are often coexistent with cellular deficiencies of potassium, low blood levels practically always indicate lack of cell potassium. This occurs when there is a drain of potassium without adequate replacement. Polyuria, such as in diabetes insipidus or in chronic glomerulonephritis, may cause potassium depletion. Even the normal daily losses in the urine can quickly lead to a severe deficiency if there is no intake of food. In addition, if potassium is lost through prolonged vomiting, diarrhea, fistulae or intestinal intubation, rapidly mounting deficits occur which may require a week to replace. Surgery, trauma or stress of any type leads to greater potassium losses both from adrenal hormone effect and from liberation of potassium from the traumatized tissue. The greatest potassium loss after surgery occurs in the first 3 days, during which the K/N ration is greater than 2.9. After this time the K^+ loss is more apt to be a starvation effect (protoplasmic loss) with a K/N ratio of 2.9. Mercurial diuretics may cause excretion of large amounts of potassium in the urine, and this loss may be even greater in salt depletion syndromes.

Rarer causes of hypokalemia are: the sudden shift of potassium from the blood into the cells such as occurs in familial periodic paralysis (this can be considered an exception to the statement that low blood levels always mean low cell levels); the excessive loss in "potassium-losing nephritis," which has been reported; Cushing's disease, in which there is an overproduction of gluco-corticoids (sugar hormone) inhibiting protein buildup, and which is associated with low serum levels of potassium; and overtreatment with cortisone or desoxycorticosterone which also causes potassium loss for the same reasons.

Although loss of intestinal juices and other causes of dehydration, diabetic acidosis and tissue anoxia lead to body potassium depletion, the blood levels may be markedly elevated, as already described. In the treatment of such a patient large quantities of glucose and water may change a high serum potassium into a hypokalemia. The potassium is diluted in the blood, excreted in the urine and shifted back into the cell, and the total body deficit rapidly becomes manifest with the clinical picture of hypopotassemia. In addition, the infusion of saline has been shown to produce a movement of potassium out of the cell (Chap. 8) and this may aggravate an existing precarious deficiency. In minor surgical procedures it has been shown that the administration of saline intravenously may cause more potassium loss than the surgical procedure itself.

FLUID SHIFT AND BLOOD PICTURE

A difference in concentration of potassium on both sides of the cell wall membrane does not provide the osmotic force in itself to initiate movements of fluid, as evidenced by the difference in concentration which normally exists. Withdrawal of potassium from the cell leads to replacement by sodium to some extent and, as far as is known, does not induce a recognizable fluid shift. The fluid dislocations which are found associated with potassium depletion are more often the cause of the potassium imbalance rather than the result. Some recent evidence has suggested that under abnormal metabolic states (i.e., cardiac decompensation) release of osmotically inactive potassium into the ionic state may cause an increase in intracellular osmolarity with resulting fluid retention and general edema (p. 131).

In untreated dehydration, even though there is an over-all potassium impoverishment, serum levels of 6 to 8 mEq./L. may be seen. Low potassium levels, less than 4 mEq./L. however, always mean potassium depletion except in familial periodic paralysis. An important laboratory method of detecting hypokalemia is the frequent coexistence of an hypochloremic alkalosis. The low chloride and elevated CO_2 are valuable evidence, especially since blood levels of potassium may be of relatively little value. The mechanism of its production is related to factors altering acid-base balance (Chap. 8).

CLINICAL PICTURE OF HYPERKALEMIA

It is the generally accepted opinion that the symptoms of potassium imbalance are primarily the result of blood levels of the ion rather than the cell content, and that these effects may be influenced also by the ratio of potassium to sodium in the blood. The exact effects of an elevated serum concentration are difficult to evaluate, since it ordinarily accompanies other profound physiologic abnormalities. Weakness of the muscles of the extremities seems to be a definite result, and listlessness, cold extremities and parasthesias may occur.

The main effects produced are upon the heart by interference with conduction through the myocardium. As a consequence bradycardia, alterations in rhythm, peripheral vascular

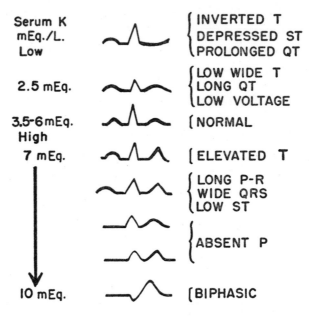

FIG. 16. Electrocardiographic changes produced by alterations in serum potassium (K) concentrations. The spreading of the QRS and lengthened QT interval in hypokalemia has been attributed to hypocalcemia rather than the hypokalemia. (Redrawn from Darrow and Pratt.)

collapse and finally cardiac arrest in diastole occur. The terminal stages appear at serum levels of 10 to 12 mEq./L.

The electrocardiogram is characteristic and may be an important method of diagnosis in the absence of blood chemical studies. The first changes (Fig. 16) are elevation of the T waves beginning at levels of 7 mEq./L.; these are best seen in the precordial leads. Spreading of the QRS then occurs with lengthening of the PR interval, and eventually the P wave disappears. Finally, a bizarre, wide QRS is produced followed by complete heart block. These progressive changes have been observed during the rapid intravenous administration of potassium solutions and are frequently recorded in the progressive intoxication of complete anuria.

Clinical Picture of Hypokalemia

To produce symptoms, the potassium deficits must be greater than the amount of K^+ which would be lost from protein breakdown. That is, cell fluid loss must have occurred over that associated with starvation without water depletion. The symptoms of hypopotassemia may be grouped into those affecting muscles, heart and intestines. The muscle weakness is progressive, as the deficiency develops, and is clinically detected by the lack of tone and the mushy feel in the large muscle groups. Reflexes become hypoactive but an actual flaccid paralysis is not common. The respiratory muscles are particularly susceptible, the patient showing signs of dyspnea, with cyanosis and respiratory failure appearing in the later stages. This has been the mode of death in some patients following treatment of diabetic coma.

In surgical patients anorexia, drowsiness and languor are early complaints starting about the fourth postoperative day. Intestinal atony and abdominal distention are a result of hypokalemia and in the postoperative patient may be mistaken for peritonitis, intestinal obstruction or prolonged postoperative ileus. The author has seen such patients treated by neostigmine and Miller-Abbott tube with no response, but immediately after potassium replacement therapy, subsidence of the distention was prompt with frequent and voluminous bowel movements.

Myocardial necrosis has been demonstrated as a result of marked potassium deficits. Cardiac dilatation and failure are the late clinical manifestations of potassium depletion, so that diagnosis should be made before these changes occur. This applies to the electrocardiographic changes as well (Fig. 16). Flattening of the T waves is the earliest change followed by depression of the S-T segment, and finally inversion of T waves. While spreading of the QRS and lengthening of the QT interval has generally been described as due to hypopotassemia, recent evidence seems to indicate that these are probably the result of an associated calcium deficiency. The suggestion has been made that increased amplitude of the U wave in the left precordial leads and fusion of the T and U waves gives the appearance of prolonged QT interval.

TREATMENT OF POTASSIUM IMBALANCE

The hyperkalemia which results from severe dehydration is corrected when fluids are replaced and rehydration is initiated; the problem, then, may quickly change to one of too low a blood concentration rather than too high. The hyperkalemia which results from inadequate urine output is more difficult to manage. Therapeutic measures designed to improve urine flow are most important, if this be accomplished. Intravenous administration of isotonic sodium chloride or sodium bicarbonate has a rapid and definite diuretic effect on potassium, but the efficacy of this depends on an adequate renal function. A diet low in protein is indicated since this presents less potassium to the patient and thereby decreases the load to be excreted. Intravenous glucose along with adequate amounts of insulin cause deposition of glycogen and potassium in the liver. The serum potassium depressing effect produced in this way thus is more prolonged. The oral administration of cation exchange resins, which do not have an added potassium cycle (p. 122), may remove appreciable amounts of this ion from the intestine, but sodium and calcium may also be lost. The use of dialysis in the treatment of hyperkalemia in renal shutdown is discussed in Chapter 12.

Hypokalemia is more amenable to preventive measures. All patients requiring parenteral fluid therapy or in whom intestinal suction is required, should routinely be given potassium-containing solutions. Patients admitted for surgery who have had prolonged vomiting or diarrhea or who show evidence of dehydration should be brought into nutritional balance and potassium should be replaced. Repeated diuresis with mercurials or other diuretics warrants careful scrutiny of the patient's diet to determine the adequacy of intake. The administration of potassium salts is indicated should these be found deficient. When the signs of hypopotassemia are evident, intravenous administration of potassium chloride, phosphate or acetate, in dilutions of 40 to 80 mEq./L. of solution, at 90 drops per minute, will rapidly correct the symptoms. The accumulated deficits can be replaced at rates which are limited by the rapidity of cell metabolism, but usually require several days for complete replacement. In addition, as much as 50 per cent of the intravenous potassium may be lost in the urine, when it is given faster than it can be assimilated. Therefore, the urinary output is not a measure of body saturation with this electrolyte. An adequate urine volume is imperative before giving potassium intravenously, since a dangerous rise in the blood level may occur quickly in the presence of oliguria or anuria.

Relationship of Potassium to Serum Calcium

It has been observed in some patients with low serum calcium that the symptoms of tetany may be obscured in the presence of a low serum potassium. Thus, in infantile diarrheas, or in patients with steatorrhea associated with low blood calcium, the administration of intravenous potassium may make a latent tetany manifest. It is not to be inferred from this that either of these substances is antidotal for the other. Calcium does not correct the EKG changes produced by hyperkalemia. The EKG picture of hypokalemia is often a combined effect of hypokalemia and hypocalcemia.

MAGNESIUM

The distribution of magnesium in body fluids resembles that of potassium, in that its position is primarily intracellular. The normal serum levels are low, averaging about 2 mEq./L. with a range of 1.4 to 2.5 mEq./L. The concentration within the cell is about 28 mEq./L., and, here, the ion apparently takes part in energy transfers involving the enzyme, adenosine triphosphate. Again, like potassium, serum levels of magnesium do not reflect the total body supply or intracellular levels of this ion. Numerous reports are present in the literature of low serum magnesium levels unassociated with any recognizable symptom complex.

The normal diet supplies about 30 mEq. (0.4 Gm.) daily, although the actual requirement is estimated to be about 18 mEq. Since the main source of supply is in the chlorophyll of green vegetables, patients on insufficient diets and with prolonged parenteral therapy may develop deficiencies of magnesium. Depletions of this ion seem to occur less readily than with potassium since the renal excretion appears to follow that of sodium. Thus, the postoperative patient tends to retain magnesium and, similarly, ACTH administration causes magnesium retention. These facts (to which there is some contradictory evidence) would seem to implicate an adrenal mechanism in the conservation of this electrolyte.

Hypermagnesemia has been reported in patients with renal insufficiency, especially where Epsom salts have been used as a laxative. In the presence of dehydration the serum levels may be elevated due to hemoconcentration, to oliguria with retention of the electrolyte and to the release of intracellular magnesium combined in cell protein. In the severe dehydrations of diabetic acidosis and infantile diarrhea, elevation of serum levels may occur despite overall body depletion. Although the clinical picture of hypermagnesemia is not well defined, lethargy, coma and respiratory failure have been reported. Whether these symptoms are due, in part, to potassium alteration is not clear.

Hypomagnesemia may result from prolonged, inadequate intake combined with continued parenteral fluid therapy. The serum levels often are below 1.4 mEq./L., and levels below 0.42 mEq./L. have been reported. Magnesium depletion has been seen following the rehydration of severely dehydrated patients with diabetic acidosis. Various convulsive states, including delirium tremens, have shown inconstantly low serum magnesium levels. In chronic alcoholism, with or without delirium tremens, low magnesium levels are fairly frequent, apparently the result of a hyponutritional state. Prolonged diuresis in congestive heart failure, and the diuretic phase of lower nephron nephrosis may cause increased magnesium loss in the urine with resulting low blood levels.

While Martin *et al.* and other researchers have been unable to identify any symptoms or signs clearly due to hypomagnesemia, Flink and his co-workers report that the most characteristic symptoms are bizarre, involuntary muscular activity appearing as gross tremors, twitching of the face and athetoid and choreiform movements of the extremities. The patient, usually quite ill, appears anxious and apprehensive, and later progresses to delirium. These workers used the patient's handwriting as a record of progress or recession of the abnormal state.

TREATMENT OF MAGNESIUM IMBALANCE

In the management of hypermagnesemia, the establishment of adequate renal flow and rehydration of the patient are most important. However, one should keep in mind that in doing this one may convert the picture to that of a deficiency pattern.

The prevention of magnesium depletion is best accomplished by using small amounts of the ion in the daily parenteral fluid. Lactated Ringer's solution and Butler's multiple electrolyte solution contain small maintenance quantities of this electrolyte (Chap. 9). In Flink's series of patients with hypomagnesemia, several showed prompt improvement with the administration of magnesium sulfate. However, many required 12 to 76 hours to correct the intracellular deficiency. Using a 50 per cent solution, 2 Gm. of magnesium sulfate are given intramuscularly 4 times daily for 3 days. In the severe cases 1 Gm. is given 4 times daily for an additional 2 to 4 days. There are no contraindications to smaller doses of magnesium sulfate, but adequate urine flow should be verified before using larger quantities.

CHAPTER EIGHT

Acid-Base Balance

Up to this point we have dealt only with the abnormalities relating to changes in the volume of fluids in the various compartments and with the osmolarity as determined primarily by the salt concentration. However, from time to time we have had to refer to changes in the ionic equilibrium also involved in the conditions which have been discussed. The changes in the relationship of cations to anions produce variations in reaction or acid-base balance of the blood. Although it is not our purpose to go into the detailed chemistry of these changes, certain simple facts must be reviewed to enable intelligent therapy.

The pH of blood serum is 7.4 and the variations of normal are between the narrow limits of 7.35 and 7.45. These are slightly on the alkaline side of electroneutrality (7.0). A shift of serum pH in the direction of 7.0 produces an acidosis, or a shift to 7.8, an alkalosis. These two extremes are near the limits of change which are compatible with life. The addition to the plasma of any acid which is highly dissociated or ionized, by supplying a greater concentration of H ions would shift the reaction to the lower pH or acid side. A weaker acid, which is less completely ionized will supply less H ions and the acid shift would be correspondingly less.

On the other hand, a solution of base, which produces a low H ion concentration, would result in a higher pH or more alkalinity. Since the normal limits of reaction in the blood are so restricted, it must be a primary concern of the body to convert strong acids or bases to less highly ionized acids and bases in order to maintain a fairly constant pH. This is accomplished by a system of buffers, of which the major ones are proteins, bicarbonates and phosphates, and also by means of the temporary shifting of electrolytes between fluid compartments. Reduced to its simplest terms, after all buffering changes have taken place, the resulting pH is dependent upon the relative amounts of carbonic acid and bicarbonate which remain in the blood, as will be shown.

As an end product of the metabolic processes, an unlimited supply of carbon dioxide is made available, which is picked up by the hemoglobin and transported to the lungs for excretion. A gradient of pressure exists from the red blood cells to the alveoli, which permits diffusion of the CO_2 from the blood to the lungs and then to the expired air. By the laws of diffusion of gasses, and as a result of their partial pressures, the fairly constant CO_2 tension in the alveoli determines the amount of carbon dioxide which is dissolved in the plasma. Increases in alveolar carbon dioxide will raise plasma CO_2; decreases, lower it. It is obvious, then, that any interference with respiration will directly affect the plasma CO_2. Likewise, any increase in the CO_2 dissolved in the plasma over that normally present will find escape by way of the alveoli.

The CO_2 dissolved in plasma combines with water to form the very weak carbonic acid, H_2CO_3. This is present in plasma mostly as the whole molecule, but a minute portion is ionized or dissociated into the hydrogen ion, H^+, and bicarbonate, HCO_3^-. The degree of this dissociation, and, therefore, the amount of hydrogen ion and pH, is definite and fixed for this substance. According to the law of "common ion effect," adding of an additional quantity of either of the ions to the solution will cause a decrease in the other by causing a shift of dissociated ions back to the whole molecular state, according to the formula

$$H_2CO_3 \rightleftharpoons [H^+][HCO_3^-]$$

Therefore, if to a solution of carbonic acid we add more HCO_3^- in the form of sodium bicarbonate, the H ion concentration drops, unionized carbonic acid increases and the solution becomes more alkaline. Or, if to the solution more carbonic acid is added, more H ions are present, the pH is lowered and the solution is more acid.

The amount of bicarbonate that is present in the plasma is not only the small amount resulting from ionization of H_2CO_3, but also the relatively large amount which is combined with the fixed cations. Increases or decreases in the total base, by increasing or decreasing the bicarbonate, cause variation in the serum pH by the common ion effect. Under ordinary conditions, most of the fixed base of the blood (Na^+, K^+ and Ca^{++}) is combined with chloride and other fixed anions (Fig. 3), except for about 27 mEq., that is available for combination with bicarbonate as base bicarbonate ($BHCO_3$). The measure of available base (also called alkali reserve) is the CO_2 combining power of the blood. In speaking of serum bicarbonate, or CO_2 combining power, we are referring, really, to the amount of base or cation that is available to combine with bicarbonate. If there is an excessive loss of Cl^-, so that more cation becomes freed, the available base becomes combined with more HCO_3^-, and the CO_2 combining power is increased. Additional bicarbonate ion is always available from carbonic acid, $HHCO_3$, and the extra H ion so freed either is taken up by other blood buffers or may shift into the cell and replace potassium there. On the other hand, if cations are lost in excess of Cl^-, there is less available base, the CO_2 combining power is decreased and the excess bicarbonate ion is excreted as carbonic acid in the urine or combined with cations (see below).

In summary, then, the reaction of the plasma depends on the relative amounts of carbonic acid and base bicarbonate, since the "common ion effect" of these substances will determine the H ion concentration and, therefore, the pH. The amount of

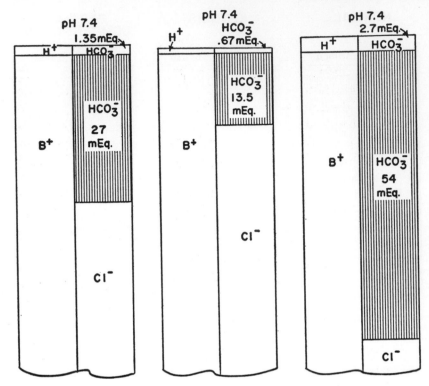

Fig. 17. Dependence of normal serum pH on a constant HHCO₃ : BHCO₃ ratio of 1:20. (*Left*) The normal concentrations of bicarbonate and carbonic acid. (*Center*) Bicarbonate is halved, as is also the carbonic acid, so that the ratio remains 1:20. The pH remains constant even though the CO₂ combining power is diminished. (*Right*) Both bicarbonate and carbonic acid are doubled, but since the ratio is still 1:20, the pH remains stationary even though the CO₂ combining power is increased.

CO₂ or carbonic acid is dependent on the lungs and normal respiration. The amount of bicarbonate depends on the amount of available base (sodium) remaining over the amount combined with the other anions. (Fig. 4).

TYPES OF ACID-BASE ABNORMALITIES

Since the pH of blood is determined by the relative amounts or ratio of HHCO₃ and BHCO₃, the usual chemical laboratory

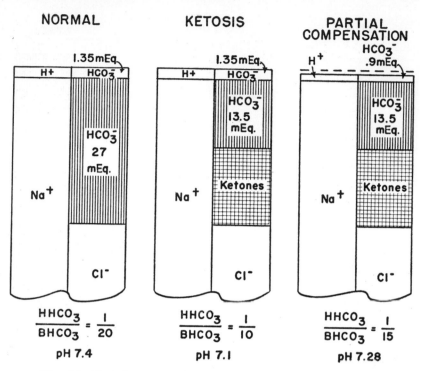

Fig. 18. Development of metabolic acidosis. (*Left*) Normal ionic equilibrium. (*Center*) Ketones accumulate at the expense of bicarbonate. The ratio is shifted in favor of carbonic acid so that an acidosis results. (*Right*) Attempt at compensation diminishes the carbonic acid. The CO_2 combining power is decreased and a less marked acidosis results.

determinations of total CO_2 or of alkali reserve, as CO_2 combining power, cannot be a measurement of blood reaction. The normal pH of 7.4 is found when the ratio of $HHCO_3$:$BHCO_3$ is 1:20. The total amount of carbonic acid or bicarbonate does not need to remain stationary; only their ratios must remain so. To clarify this relationship, note in Figure 17 that normally there are 1.35 mEq. or 3 volumes per cent of $HHCO_3$ to 27 mEq. or 60 volumes per cent of $BHCO_3$. This is the ratio of 1:20, and at this ratio the pH is 7.4. If the concentration of $BHCO_3$ is halved to 13.5 mEq., to maintain a ratio of 1:20 and a pH of 7.4, $HHCO_3$ must also be halved to .67 mEq. Or, if

$BHCO_3$ is doubled to 54 mEq., the $HHCO_3$ must also be doubled to 2.7 mEq., to maintain a pH of 7.4.

The great changes of bicarbonate necessary to offset small variations in a concentration of H_2CO_3 at this pH range are quite evident. Under conditions of alteration of either carbonic acid or bicarbonate, the body attempts to correct the deviation by a compensatory change in the other. If the correction is complete so that the normal pH results it is spoken of as a "compensated change." More often, however, the correction falls short of complete compensation and it is then referred to as an "uncompensated change."

METABOLIC ACIDOSIS

To illustrate this let us assume that we have a diabetic patient who begins to accumulate ketonic acids in the blood due to insufficient insulin (Fig. 18). These act as additional anions in the plasma to bind some of the base which has been in combination with bicarbonate. The displaced bicarbonate ion is buffered and finally the serum bicarbonate level is halved. The ratio is now in favor of $HHCO_3$, so that an acidosis has been produced. In the attempt to correct this change, there occurs an increase in respiratory volume induced by the effect of acidosis on the respiratory centers (acidotic breathing) so that more CO_2 is eliminated, thereby tending to restore the normal balance. This is accomplished to some extent, so that the ratio is improved but still in favor of $HHCO_3$. The pH remains low; this is referred to as an uncompensated metabolic acidosis. The CO_2 combining power will be found to be less than its normal 27 mEq./L. It is felt by some that there can never be complete compensation in these cases since the hyperpnea resulting from the acidosis becomes less as the acidosis improves, so that the stimulus for the correction disappears before compensation is complete. For this reason, perhaps a better term would be a "partially compensated" metabolic acidosis. It should be noted that this is a metabolic change in reaction, in which the initial alteration occurred in the amount of bicarbonate, with the carbonic acid then adjusted to this.

Metabolic acidosis is found whenever available base is decreased, although the total base remains unchanged, as in starvation where ketones increase in the blood in a manner similar to that described above. In kidney failure or uremia, the retention of the anions, phosphate and sulfate, also decreases available base. Large doses of acidifying salts, such as ammonium chloride, leave an excess of chloride ion when metabolized while the ammonia is converted to urea in the liver. Excessive exercise or anoxia leads to an accumulation of organic acids at the expense of bicarbonate. Metabolic acidosis may result also from excessive loss of base without equivalent loss of chloride, as in the diarrheas, so there is a relative chloride excess. The treatment of acidosis necessitates the removal of the excess anions (chloride, ketones, etc.) or replacement of the lost base thus making more available for combination with HCO_3^-.

METABOLIC ALKALOSIS

Let us now assume we have a patient who is vomiting and losing large amounts of chloride as compared to smaller amounts of sodium (Fig. 19). As the serum chloride is decreased, more sodium is left unattached and available to combine with bicarbonate. In the diagram, bicarbonate is doubled in amount with the ionic balance now in favor of the bicarbonate so that an alkalosis results. Compensation is attempted by a diminished respiratory exchange and H_2CO_3 is retained. Again, this is not accomplished completely so that the ratio, although improved, remains in favor of bicarbonate and the pH is increased. An uncompensated metabolic alkalosis results and the CO_2 combining power is increased above its normal value. Here again, the primary change is a metabolic one, the first alteration occurring in the bicarbonate with a compensatory effect on the H_2CO_3.

Metabolic alkalosis is found when HCO_3^-, or alkali reserve, is increased although the total base remains unchanged. This occurs in practice when excess chlorides have been removed by excessive vomiting or gastric suction without replace-

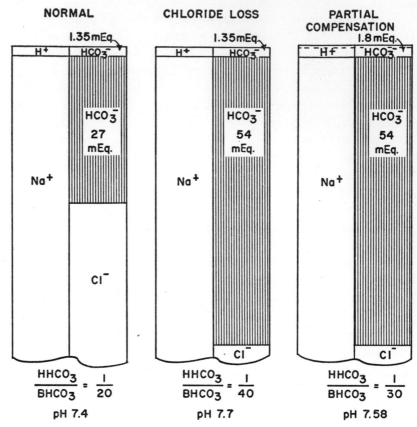

FIG. 19. Development of metabolic alkalosis. (*Left*) Normal
state. (*Center*) Chlorides have been lost with a resulting increase in alkali reserve or bicarbonate. The ratio, now in favor
of bicarbonate, consequently produces an alkalosis. (*Right*) Attempt at compensation increases the carbonic acid. A less
marked alkalosis results and the CO_2 combining power is
increased.

ment of electrolytes; or by too vigorous intestinal irrigation through indwelling tubes. Administration of large
doses of alkali (soda bicarbonate) increases available base
over anions and results in metabolic alkalosis. In the
presence of cellular potassium depletion, alkalosis develops
with an elevated bicarbonate and a lowered serum chloride,
making this an important means of detecting potassium deficit

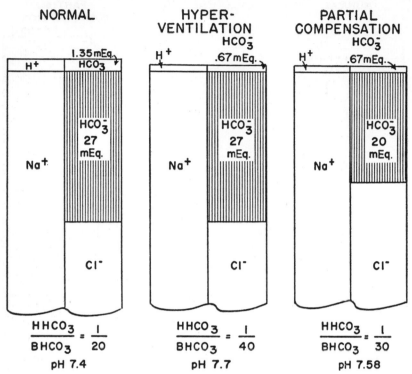

FIG. 20. Development of respiratory alkalosis. (*Left*) The normal ratio of carbonic acid and bicarbonate. (*Center*) Hyperventilation has decreased the carbonic acid leaving a relative preponderance of bicarbonate and an alkalosis. (*Right*) Partial compensation takes place by decrease in bicarbonate with a lowered CO_2 combining power, although there is still an alkalosis.

(see below). Cushing's disease with potassium deficit produces a similar picture. Treatment of the alkalosis requires replacing the lost anions to diminish available base, or to replace the deficient potassium.

Respiratory Alkalosis

Now let us assume the case of a nervous patient who is breathing deeply and rapidly as the result of some frightening symptom or situation. The increased ventilation blows off unusually large amounts of CO_2 so that the alveolar partial

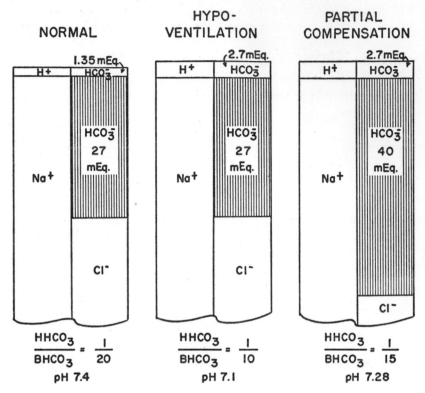

Fig. 21. Development of respiratory acidosis. (*Left*) The normal state. (*Center*) Interference with the excretion of CO_2 gives an increased concentration of carbonic acid and an acidosis. (*Right*) Compensation partially corrects the ratio by increasing bicarbonate. An elevated CO_2 combining power results although an acidosis still persists.

pressure and the plasma carbonic acid concentration is decreased by half (Fig. 20). The proportion of $HHCO_3$ to $BHCO_3$ is now diminished as to carbonic acid so that the H ion concentration is lowered with a resulting alkalosis. To correct the imbalance the kidneys begin to excrete more bicarbonate. Ordinarily this effort improves the ratio, although not completely, and the shift remains in favor of bicarbonate, giving an uncompensated respiratory alkalosis. The CO_2 combining power, however, is *lowered*. This differs from the previous imbalances in that the initiating fault is in the respiratory control and the bicarbonate change is the secondary effect. A low carbon dioxide combining power in the presence of an alkalosis is the result.

Respiratory alkalosis occurs in any condition causing hyperventilation, where this is not the result of interference with gaseous exchange in the lungs. It may be seen in high fevers, central nervous system lesions and in the anoxia of the cardiac or of high altitudes. Treatment of this alkalosis is accomplished by preventing CO_2 loss by slowing respiration or by administering CO_2 gas by mask.

RESPIRATORY ACIDOSIS

Let us take now a patient with advanced emphysema who has marked impairment of respiratory movements and a diminished tidal air volume. Inadequate exchange of gasses in the lung causes a retention of carbon dioxide, and carbonic acid concentration, therefore, increases in the blood serum (Fig. 21). The ratio of $HHCO_3$ to $BHCO_3$ now favors the carbonic acid, thereby producing an elevated H ion concentration and acidosis. The kidneys attempt to readjust by excreting more ammonium and chloride, thus conserving more fixed cations in the plasma to form bicarbonate. This attempt at adjustment frequently is incomplete and the ratio still favors $HHCO_3$ with a lowered pH. An uncompensated respiratory acidosis is the result, but the CO_2 combining power is *elevated*.

Respiratory acidosis occurs in any condition where there is interference with the exchange of gasses within the lung so that CO_2 is not adequately blown off. This may happen in marked narcosis from drugs, especially narcotics, central nervous system depression from any cause, emphysema and bronchiectasis. Paralysis of respiration in poliomyelitis inevitably leads to respiratory acidosis and is one of the major problems in the management of respirator cases.

Aggravation of the respiratory acidosis in emphysematous patients, when these individuals are placed in high concentrations of oxygen, can produce alarming symptoms leading to death. The mechanism is believed to be the result of the sudden removal of the respiratory stimulation induced by the chronic anoxemia, thereby causing depression of respiration with even greater retention of CO_2 and an accentuation of the acidosis. Besides its effects on pH, the high CO_2 concentration also contributes to the final narcosis. As chemical adjustment to the acidosis becomes partially compensated, a very high CO_2 combining power may be found, but the pH may be normal or very nearly so (Table 3). Under these conditions

DATE	TOTAL CO_2 VOL. %	SERUM pH
9-21	62.6	7.4
9-28	Oxygen room—	50% oxygen
10-2	90.1	7.38
10-6	93.7	
10-19	91.7	7.32
10-20	Oxygen tent	35% or less O_2
11-6	68.9	7.46
11-9	72.2	
12-5	66.8	

TABLE 3. Effect of oxygen therapy on serum pH in patient with pulmonary fibrosis. The marked increase in CO_2 retention and corresponding drop in pH is clearly shown when high concentrations of oxygen are administered with respiratory acidosis. (Data from Richards)

it becomes a problem to remove these patients from the oxygen since they will develop a respiratory alkalosis which may be just as troublesome. A type of physiologic addiction to the high concentration of oxygen has developed. Treatment of respiratory acidosis requires more efficient removal of CO_2 by improvement of gaseous exchange. The symptoms of marked acidosis require increasing available base by the cautious adding of more bicarbonate or by increasing the loss of fixed anions. The value of the carbonic anhydrase inhibitor, Diamox, in treatment of respiratory acidosis remains to be determined. Some evidence seems to indicate that respiratory elimination of CO_2 may be improved with this drug. (See p. 124)

DIAGNOSIS AND DIFFERENTIAL DIAGNOSIS

Acidosis or alkalosis is practically always associated with some major fluid imbalance, thus making difficult the delineation of the symptoms of acid-base imbalance from those of severe dehydration, salt depletion or potassium deficit. In acidosis the skin may be flushed and warm and there may be hyperpneic breathing. The air hunger of diabetic acidosis is characteristic and in the presence of ketones one finds the typical acetone breath. Variation in the depth or rate of respiration is not diagnostic, however, since one may find hyperpnea in a patient who has a respiratory alkalosis. The progressive picture of acidosis is ordinarily part of the dehydration, hyperkalemia and shock which are usually associated with it. Metabolic alkalosis produces few symptoms except, possibly, a slow, shallow respiration. Increased muscular irritability may result in tetany (hyperventilation tetany) which is identical in appearance to that due to hypocalcemia.

The CO_2 combining power of the blood, which measures available alkali, or alkali reserve, does not distinguish, in itself, between acidosis or alkalosis. By separately measuring both bicarbonate and carbonic acid, the H ion concentration or pH can be determined from the quantitative relationship. To determine accurately the type of imbalance and the degree of compensation which has taken place, total CO_2 and pH are required. In spite of this, in many clinical situations the physician can fairly well determine the change in reaction from a careful evaluation of the patient, aided by a determination of the CO_2 combining power. If serum sodium, total base or chloride can also be obtained, the diagnosis becomes much easier. For example, a low CO_2 combining power in the presence of known diabetes, severe renal disease or associated with dehydration postoperatively are very likely to be metabolic in origin. On the other hand, CO_2 changes in the presence of major lung pathology or disease interfering with respiration are apt to be of respiratory origin. Where both metabolic and respiratory factors are prominent features of the disease, the chemical determination is the only means of differentiating alkalosis from acidosis.

ELECTROLYTE SHIFTS IN ACIDOSIS AND ALKALOSIS

Darrow's studies on the composition of intracellular fluids have done much to explain some of the observed peculiarities of serum electrolyte composition in various disease states. It was pointed out in Figure 3 that the sodium concentration within the cell bears a definite relationship to the extracellular bicarbonate concentration. In any pathologic state, which results in a metabolic alkalosis with increase in serum bicarbonate, there is a transfer of sodium into the cell. By making less base available, this helps to reduce the amount of bicarbonate and, hence, ameliorates the severity of the alkalosis. This is in effect, then, an additional buffer mechanism for blood pH. Coincident with this intracellular shift, there is a movement of potassium out of the cell, the quantity of which is greater than the amount of sodium which moved in. In general, although not always, there seems to be a reciprocal relationship between intracellular sodium and potassium so that under abnormal conditions as much as 75 mEq./L. of potassium may be replaced by 50 mEq./L. of sodium. When one considers the actual total volume of intracellular fluid in the body this amount of sodium becomes quite considerable. In metabolic alkalosis the difference between the potassium lost and the sodium gained in the cell, is made up by an intracellular movement of H ions, which have been freed from the H_2CO_3 as the HCO_3 ion takes part in the developing alkalosis. Thus, an extracellular alkalosis is accompanied by an intracellular acidosis. The dislodged K ion is excreted as KCl, and the serum chloride level drops. This may be diagramed:

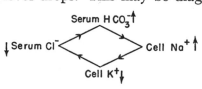

The above shifts apparently represent a state of biologic equilibrium, so that these movements of ions between fluid compartments will take place regardless of which of the electrolytes concentration is altered first. For example, in a patient who is vomiting and losing large amounts of chloride, the serum chloride drops, bicarbonate increases, sodium moves intracellularly and potassium moves out. Or, if, during severe dehydration or starvation, large amounts of potassium are lost, the final picture is the same. Clinically, therefore, the presence of a hypochloremic alkalosis (serum chloride lowered, CO_2 combining power elevated) will perpetuate itself until both the deficient substances are replaced, that is, chloride and potassium. Replacement of one alone will not correct the alkalosis. These relationships are a biologic adjustment rather than a chemical one, since several days are required both for their development and correction. Why the kidney does not correct the alkalosis in the presence of only the potassium deficit is not known. As long as the potassium deficit exists, the kidney will not excrete sodium to reduce available base, and administration of large doses of chloride, as ammonium chloride, will not correct the alkalosis until sufficient potassium is also replaced. In the discussion dealing with potassium abnormalities (Chap. 7) were listed the causes of potassium depletion. These may all contribute to the production of hypochloremic alkalosis. Intravenous administration of saline has been shown to diurese large amounts of potassium as the sodium is deposited in the cell. It is well to recognize that sodium cannot replace the metabolic function of potassium and the presence of sodium in the cell does not compensate for loss of the normal intracellular cation.

In metabolic acidosis, on the other hand, an opposite movement occurs. In the steady state here, serum chloride increases with a corresponding drop in bicarbonate. Sodium moves out of the cell making more base available, and again acting as a buffer mechanism. Potassium should increase in the cell according to the diagram:

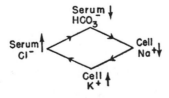

Actually, however, those clinical states which lead to acidosis, such as diabetes, diarrhea or starvation, are all accompanied by protein breakdown and cell fluid loss. As a result, potassium is lost in large quantities along with the cell sodium. In fact, a number of studies have shown that these patients may even have a shift of sodium into the cell to partially replace the lost potassium. Therefore, in a patient with severe diarrhea, who is losing sodium in the stool, added sodium depletion may result from intracellular movement of this electrolyte. It is evident from this, that measurement of serum sodium in acidosis does not accurately picture the total sodium loss, since the cell sodium may be elevated. On the other hand, very large cellular deficits may exist. Theoretically, although cell potassium should be elevated, the replacement with sodium chloride alone in the treatment of these patients converts the multiple deficiency into a potassium deficiency and a metabolic alkalosis results. These intracellular and extracellular potassium-sodium shifts are not merely the substitution of one ion for the other, but are the result of metabolic changes and oxygen utilization. For this reason, the shifts which occur are not quantitatively predictable from measurement of extracellular fluid electrolyte changes.

Recent studies on the movement of electrolytes in respiratory acidosis and alkalosis have shown that the shifts are not as marked as in those of metabolic origin. In many instances no intracellular changes could be demonstrated. Where changes did occur within the cell they were in line with what might be expected from the serum pH and were not related to the amount of serum bicarbonate or the partial pressure of CO_2.

RENAL REGULATION OF ACID-BASE BALANCE

Although respiration plays an important role in maintaining the normal reaction of blood by excreting CO_2, the ultimate correction of the ionic imbalances resides in renal control. From the practical therapeutic point of view, the physician can do more towards management by directing efforts at improving kidney regulation than is possible in respiratory control.

During the normal processes of metabolism, the acid radicals, PO_4^{--} and SO_4^{--}, are formed in large quantities and transported to the kidneys combined as sodium salts in the blood. If these were to be excreted in the urine still bound to sodium, depletions of this cation would rapidly occur.

Under conditions of normal blood pH, with an alkali reserve or bicarbonate of 27 mEq./L., little base is excreted in the urine. If a metabolic acidosis develops with a diminished alkali reserve, base is reabsorbed by the kidney tubules, leaving a more acid urine. If the alkali reserve is elevated with an alkalosis, more bicarbonate-bound base is excreted, and the urine becomes more alkaline. An exception to this occurs in the presence of low serum chloride (hypochloremic alkalosis with sodium depletion) and with hyperventilation, under which circumstances bicarbonate-bound base is reabsorbed in conserving the base, leaving an acid urine in spite of a serum alkalosis. In respiratory acidosis more NH_4^+ is excreted, thus conserving fixed base. Pitts feels that the renal control of bicarbonate-bound base reabsorption is more a function of CO_2 tension in the blood rather than pH.

Base Conservation

The reabsorption of fixed cations which are bound to excretable anions can be accomplished only by a mechanism in which some other ions can be supplied to replace them. The first of these is the exchange replacement of sodium or other base by the H ion supplied from the tubules. The H^+ is liberated by the ionization of carbonic acid into H^+ and HCO_3^-, and the sodium of the glomerular filtrate is reabsorbed and bound to the bicarbonate ion. The formation of the carbonic acid from H_2O and CO_2 depends on the presence of the enzyme, carbonic anhydrase. Blocking the action of this substance will prevent the formation of $HHCO_3$ and the subsequent H ion release; this principle is applied in the clinical use of certain diuretic substances (such as Diamox). The measurement of this base conservation, which is called the "titratable acid" determines the difference in H ion concentration between serum and the excreted urine. An example of base conserva-

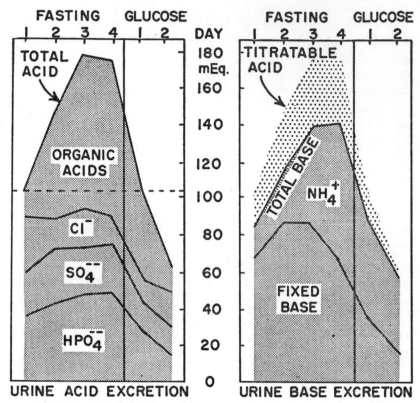

FIG. 22. Conservation of fixed base in the excretion of excess
"acid radicals." (*Left*) During the fasting state the production
of ketones and increased amounts of sulfates and phosphates
increase the total acid for excretion above the prefasting level,
which is represented by the dotted horizontal line. With the
administration of glucose the acid excretion rapidly abates.
(*Right*) At the onset of the fasting state some acids are covered
by fixed base, but the base excretion decreases as the ammonium production of the kidney increases. Additional base is
saved by excreting a more acid urine (lower pH). This is called
the "titratable acid." (From Gamble)

tion by this means is the conversion of dibasic phosphate,
B_2HPO_4, and its excretion as monobasic phosphate, BH_2PO_4.

The second method of base conservation is in the production of the ammonium ion, by the kidney tubules, from amino
acids, especially glutamine (Fig. 22). This is deaminified in

the tubule cells and the NH_3 then is available to replace base and combine with the excreted anion. In the process of becoming a salt the NH_3 takes on another H ion from the carbonic acid to form NH_4^+, so that interference with H ion production also interferes with the ammonium mechanism for base conservation. When the need for base conservation exceeds that which is accomplished by increasing titratable acidity, increasing amounts of NH_4^+ are liberated. About 4 days are required for the maximum efficiency of NH_4^+ production to develop. Severe tubular damage, as in chronic nephritis, impairs the ability to produce NH_4^+ to the extent that fixed base cannot be conserved. By the H ion exchange and ammonium production the kidney is able to convert a glomerular filtrate with a pH of 7.4 into urine with a pH as low as 4.5, which is the limit of urine acidity.

With base conservation functioning to capacity, if there is still excess anion to be excreted, or in the excretion of Cl^- or SO_4^{--}, which form strong acids, fixed base such as Na^+, Ca^{++} and K^+ must be used. Excessive sodium lost in this way may appreciably deplete the serum of sodium. In chronic nephritis, where NH_4^+ production is greatly impaired, patients may develop what has been called a "salt-losing nephritis." In severe renal disease in children, by the same means, large amounts of calcium may be lost producing the picture of "renal rickets." In adults, the equivalent process causes renal osteomalacia. Recently, a "potassium-losing nephritis" was reported in which this cation is used to cover loss of anion, with a resulting hypokalemia. The loss of the different ions depends on their availability and, possibly, on some transport factors within the tubule cells.

The administration of acidifying salts as diuretics makes use of the NH_4^+ producing property of the kidney. The diuretic, ammonium chloride, actually supplies excess anions, since the ammonium is converted to urea in the liver, leaving the Cl ion to be excreted. For the first 4 days, until NH_4^+ production by the tubules has reached its peak, body sodium is used to cover the excretion of the chloride. After this time, the production of NH_4^+ has reached a point where sodium is being well protected, (Fig. 22). For this reason administration of ammonium chloride for longer than a 4-day period serves no practical purpose. In chronic nephritis, where the ability to produce ammonia is lost, continuous administration of acidifying salts will cause continuous loss of fixed base, resulting in sodium depletion, chloride retention and a metabolic acidosis.

CONSERVATION OF ANIONS

A similar mechanism functions for the relatively few instances where the number of base radicals to be excreted is in excess of the acid. In order that acid-base balance be maintained, chloride cannot be used for this purpose to any great extent. The kidneys may conserve chloride to a small degree by excreting a urine which is more alkaline (up to pH 7.8) than serum. This can be called "titratable alkali."

Most important is the increase in excretion of base as bicarbonate in the urine. The HCO_3 ion is supplied by the tubules and is readily available to cover loss of cations, thus sparing chloride. It is evident from this that normal kidneys, given adequate fluid to permit the manipulations of the electrolytes, can do a remarkable job of balancing electrolytes and maintaining a normal pH.

ACID-BASE CHANGES IN CLINICAL STATES

There is no exact picture of serum electrolyte structure that can be predicted for any given clinical situation because of the interplay of so many variable factors. Examining some representative cases will give a better conception of the abnormalities which occur in the serum chemistries and the factors involved in their production. It will be recalled in Figure 4 that the total number of anions must equal the total cations, so that variations in total base, which is primarily sodium, will cause corresponding variations in total acids.

VOMITING, GASTRIC LAVAGE AND PYLORIC OBSTRUCTION

In Figure 23, loss of Cl^- occurs in excess of sodium so that a lowered serum chloride results with a compensatory increase in bicarbonate. In spite of the loss of hypotonic secretions,

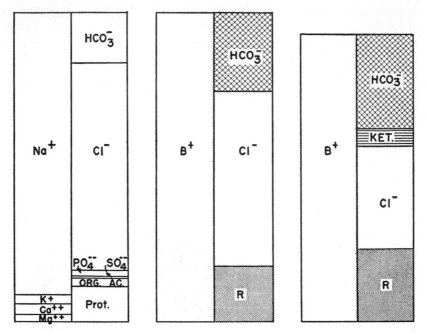

Fɪɢ. 23. Serum electrolytes in vomiting, gastric suction and pyloric obstruction. (*Left*) The normal electrolyte pattern. (*Center*) Loss of chloride results in an increased CO_2 combining power. Phosphates, sulfates, organic acids and proteins are shown as R. (*Right*) With continued electrolyte loss the concentration of base (B^+) decreases and with it blood volume diminishes. The concentration of proteins so produced, and the diminished renal blood flow, resulting in retention of PO_4 and SO_4, causes an increase in R. With inadequate caloric intake ketones appear, and a ketosis exists in the presence of an alkalosis.

which would tend to cause hypertonicity, the normal concentration of sodium is maintained early by renal correction with the excretion of sodium bicarbonate in an alkaline urine. The picture therefore is a metabolic alkalosis (center) with a low serum chloride, an elevated CO_2 combining power, and a normal sodium concentration, although blood volume is now contracted. Attempts now are made to maintain blood volume in spite of sodium loss, resulting in a picture of salt depletion also, with diminished total base concentration, especially if

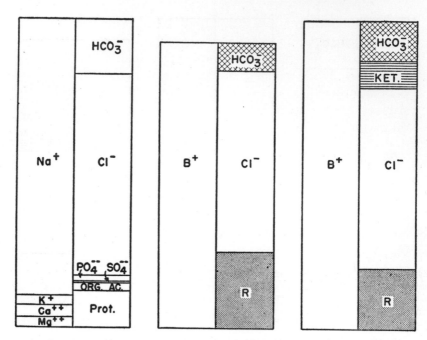

Fɪɢ. 24. Serum electrolytes in diarrhea and fasting. (*Left*)
The normal electrolyte pattern. (*Center*) Loss of base (B⁺)
results in a diminished sodium concentration and also a diminished alkali reserve or CO_2 combining power. Impaired renal
function with retention of phosphates, sulfates and organic
acids, and protein concentration cause an increase of R.
(*Right*) In fasting, accumulation of ketones decreases the available base, and CO_2 combining power is diminished with a
metabolic acidosis.

there has been continued water replacement. At this stage
(right) there is the added factor of low blood volume and
sodium depletion with concentration of the plasma protein.
Sodium conservation at this stage results in an acid urine in
spite of blood alkalosis. Impairment of kidney function is the
result of diminished blood flow, with retention of organic acids,
phosphates and sulfates occurring. These increase in the
serum along with protein. Both are shown in the diagram as
R. The intracellular changes associated with the alkalosis are
an acidosis with increase in cell sodium and loss of potassium.

Treatment requires replacement of blood volume with fluids to establish renal flow and the correction of the salt depletion to maintain the blood volume. The alkalosis can be corrected by supplying additional chloride and potassium. If potassium is not replaced, biologic equilibria will cause a persistence of the alkalosis in spite of adequate chloride and sodium administration.

DIARRHEA, INTESTINAL SUCTION AND FISTULA

Loss of sodium occurs in excess of chloride in an isotonic or hypertonic secretion (Fig. 24). Since the total sodium concentration is diminished (center), there is a contraction of the blood volume and diminution of renal blood flow. These factors result in a concentration of protein and retention of organic acids, phosphates and sulfates with an elevation of R in the diagram. The picture is that of a metabolic acidosis, and, as far as chloride and CO_2 combining power are concerned, there is a marked decrease in both but a proportionately greater loss of the bicarbonate. The concurrent intracellular changes would be either an increase or decrease of sodium, but practically always a diminished cellular potassium due to loss of this ion in the intestinal secretion. Treatment requires adequate fluid, sodium chloride, bicarbonate and potassium. The result of failure in replacing potassium would be a conversion of the acidosis to an alkalosis.

FASTING AND STARVATION

In the absence of adequate carbohydrate ingestion, fats are utilized in large amounts for caloric requirements with production of excessive amounts of ketonic acids (Fig. 24). These increase in the blood, displacing bicarbonate from available base and an acidosis results (right). The ketones, being strong acids, are excreted in combination with fixed base by the kidneys. Intracellular changes in starvation result in protein breakdown and potassium loss. Treatment consists of administration of glucose to prevent ketone formation. Sodium lactate replaces lost fixed base without adding more anions (lactate metabolizes into CO_2 and water).

It might be well to point out here that in the development of acid-base imbalances, there is almost always disparity in the loss of sodium and chloride in the urine. For this reason measurement of chloride output in the urine does not accurately measure sodium loss. Serum levels of chloride are certainly misleading when used for estimating serum sodium. The total of chloride and bicarbonate likewise will not measure sodium if ketones, phosphates or sulfates are increased.

Considerable alteration in the balance of electrolytes may result from the contraction of blood volume in dehydration. Not infrequently the mere replacement of salt and fluids, by correcting dehydration and improving kidney function, will in itself repair an existing imbalance in acid-base relationship. In treatment, therefore, attention should be given first to replacement of fluid to insure an adequate urine volume, before specific efforts are made at correction of acid-base imbalance.

CHAPTER NINE

Treatment of the
Major Depletions

With an understanding of the foregoing physiologic principles as a basis, the therapy of the complex depletions should
be logical and effective. However, too often there is the temp-
tation to treat the blood electrolyte level with a failure to take
into consideration the whole clinical picture. As Mudge has
stated, one should not ask, in the face of an abnormal electrolyte determination, "How do we get this back to normal?," but
rather "What harm is this doing the patient?" Vigorous treatment of chronic imbalances may lead to correction of the
chemistry but worsening of the clinical state. Abnormalities
which are acutely developed are more responsive to vigorous
therapy.

The existing abnormalities in any patient should be determined and expressed in terms of volume deficit, osmolarity
and acid-base imbalance. The solutions used in therapy will
produce their effects in these three directions and the choice
of the proper agent depends upon which effect is desired.
Table 4 lists the most generally available solutions commer-
cially and their chemical composition.

TABLE 4. ELECTROLYTE COMPOSITION OF COMMONLY USED REPAIR SOLUTIONS

	Na mEq./L.	K mEq./L.	Cl mEq./L.	HCO_3 mEq./L.	Other mEq./L.
Isotonic NaCl 0.9%	155		155		
Hypotonic NaCl 0.45%	77		77		
Hypertonic NaCl					
5%	860		860		
3%	520		520		
M/6 Sodium Lactate	166			166	
Hartmann's Lactated Ringer's..	130	5	118	25	Calcium - 3 Magnesium - 2
Darrow's "K Lactate"	120	35	105	50	
Butler's Multiple Electrolyte Solution (approx.) ...	42	30	35	25	PO_4 - 16 Magnesium - 5
Potassium Chloride amp..		20	20		
Potassium Chloride amp..		40	40		
Ammonium Chloride 0.9%..			167		Ammonium - 167
Blood Plasma ...	142	5	103	27	

SOLUTIONS AVAILABLE FOR TREATMENT

Sodium Chloride 0.9 per cent. Being isotonic with blood, this solution restores extracellular fluid volume and dilutes the cells and other constituents of blood. It will have no immediate effect in changing osmolarity or sodium concentration of the blood since it does not supply extra sodium above the normal levels of concentration. Over a period of time, however, the salt so administered will be utilized to replace the deficits. This solution supplies chloride ions in excess of sodium as compared to blood serum concentration and therefore tends to produce a hyperchloremic acidosis. It is ordinarily administered at a rate of 400 cc. per hour, although it may be given as fast as 2,000 cc. per hour in patients without cardiovascular impairment who are badly dehydrated.

Hypotonic Saline, 0.45 per cent. Since water is present in excess of salt in this solution, water is made immediately available for excretory needs, and at the same time the amount of salt necessary for daily requirements is supplied. It is especially useful for daily maintenance but is of less value for replacement of deficits. The excess chloride over the sodium has a slight tendency to cause acidosis of rather insignificant proportions, if there is no pre-existing acid-base imbalance.

Three per cent and 5 per cent Sodium Chloride. These hypertonic saline solutions are especially valuable for the treatment of salt depletion since the bulk of the salt in these solutions is immediately available for raising the osmolarity of the blood. Identical amounts of salt given as normal saline would introduce dangerously large amounts of fluid into the vascular compartment. Rates of administration should not be more than 200 cc. per hour. One should not give more than 400 cc. of the 5 per cent solution at one time without re-evaluating the patient's need for more.

One Sixth Molar (M/6) Sodium Lactate. This solution is also isotonic, supplying sodium without chloride. The lactate, having some caloric value, is metabolized into carbonic acid and quickly excreted leaving the sodium ion free to augment the available base and thereby tending to produce an alkalosis. Since the sodium is isosmotic with blood serum it is not immediately available to increase osmolarity of blood. In the treatment of acidosis, one third of the total amount of sodium administered may be given as the lactate. Rarely is more than this amount required.

Hartmann's Lactated Ringer's Solution. This solution most nearly resembles the electrolytic structure of normal blood serum. Since there is no excess of chloride or bicarbonate, no change in reaction of the blood is induced. The amount of potassium present is not sufficient for daily potassium maintenance and certainly not for replacement of existing potassium deficits. A small amount of calcium is also present in this solution.

Darrow's "K Lactate" Solution. This contains sodium and chloride in the normal serum ratio and, in addition, has in each liter the amount of potassium required to replace the usual daily loss. For postoperative or post-traumatic use, the amount of sodium is greater than required unless other sources of sodium loss exist. It may be given intravenously or subcutaneously if the proper precautions are exercised for administering potassium solution. It has been primarily used for the treatment of infantile diarrhea and diabetic acidosis.

Butler's Multiple Electrolyte Solution. This is a hypotonic solution which supplies the daily ordinary requirement of salt. Potassium is also present in the amount normally lost each day, and it also supplies the intracellular electrolytes, phosphate and magnesium. Originally it was used in the treatment of diabetic acidosis, but has been applied to other types of dehydration as well. Commercial preparations resembling this combination are now available.

Potassium Chloride. Ampules of 20 mEq. and of 40 mEq. of potassium chloride may be added to 5 per cent glucose solutions or other electrolyte solutions for maintenance and replacement of potassium deficits. No more than 40 mEq. should be given in 1 L. of intravenous solution administered at about 90 drops per minute, or 400 cc. per hour, observing the proper precautions. It is probably inadvisable to administer more than 120 mEq. intravenously daily unless the effects are checked by frequent examinations and electrocardiographic tracings. Potassium is present in other electrolyte solutions in therapeutic quantities and requires the same precautions in administration.

Five per cent Glucose in Water. Although isotonic when administered, the metabolism of the glucose (200 Cal. per L.) leaves only water which is available for rehydration and for excretory purposes. Given intravenously it may cause some sodium loss in the urine. For the utilization of administered potassium adequate amounts of glucose must also be given, so that this solution makes a good vehicle for intravenous potassium solution. When given by hypodermoclysis, sodium chloride will diffuse into it from the surrounding tissues and blood, thus seriously aggravating an already existing salt depletion.

Ammonium Chloride. Since the NH_4^+ is metabolized by the liver, this solution leaves free chloride ions, and, thus, is used in alkalosis with marked hypochloremia. The indications for its use are not commonly encountered.

Plasma Expanders. Dextran is a carbohydrate of high molecular weight, forming a colloidal suspension with physical properties similar to plasma. It is given in quantities of 500 cc. of the 6 per cent solution, either with or without 0.9 per cent saline. While from 25 to 40 per cent is excreted by way of the kidneys in the first 24 hours, it is believed that most of that which remains is slowly metabolized and utilized by the body. The colloidal osmotic effect causes an increase in blood volume and makes the substance especially valuable for the treatment of shock of neurogenic or traumatic origin. It does not replace blood in hemorrhage, but does have an advantage over plasma in that it does not carry the virus of homologous serum hepatitis. It has also been used in the treatment of burns, and in the salt-free solution, for hypoalbuminemic edema. Since the protein level is unaffected by this substance, its value in edema is only transitory. Mild allergic reactions have been reported. Other plasma expanders with similar properties are available.

Other Electrolyte Solutions. Many solutions containing various combinations of electrolytes have been prepared and many of these are now available in already mixed form from the commercial drug houses. Some are designed to replace gastric juice loss while others are used for duodenal and intestinal losses. Solutions containing glucose, invert sugar and amino acids are supplied in various combinations with electrolyte solutions, for caloric value and protein-building effects. Each of these prepared solutions has its own particular field of usefulness and the reader at this stage should be able to evaluate its relative merits. Solutions for routine postoperative replacement have been suggested by Elman and by Fox and their associates, and others. These are applicable, of course, only where usual losses occur. The complicating factors of intestinal intubation or fistulae make the use of routine solutions hazardous. A routine solution can no more be used for maintaining fluid balance than can a routine diet maintain all diabetics.

Order of Administration

The first step in treatment should be the reconstitution of the extracellular fluid and blood volume. This is accomplished best by isotonic saline, lactated Ringer's or M/6 sodium lactate. With these, fluid is made available for increasing the volume of urine. To this same end one can never err by giving whole plasma or blood which dilutes the hemoconcentration, raises blood pressure and establishes renal flow. Glucose in water, although isotonic when administered, has little effect in increasing blood volume since the glucose is rapidly utilized. As blood volume is being restored, attention is then directed to the osmolar changes and the hypertonicity or hypotonicity is corrected. In primary water depletion with hypertonicity of the blood, 5 per cent glucose in water serves well. In salt depletion, however, this glucose solution even though isotonic will aggravate the hyponatremia both by dilution of the blood and by its salt-diuresing effect. For these reasons salt depletion requires the administration of saline solution before water or other hypotonic solutions.

It has been shown that gross water deficits, by impairment of kidney function, can in itself cause a metabolic acidosis through retention of acid radicals; or by cell damage, a hypokalemic alkalosis. Correction of volume deficits and osmolarity, by improving renal function, will in itself often right an acid-base imbalance. However, this may be aided by supplying the solution which tends to correct the existing ionic imbalance; sodium chloride can be used for alkalosis and M/6 sodium lactate for acidosis.

TREATMENT OF WATER DEPLETION

The representative cases presented below are meant only to indicate the approach to proper therapy. Each case must be analyzed on its own merits and treatment prescribed accordingly. Other means of determining the deficits may be equally as good, and the treatments indicated could be varied in many ways.

The estimation of the amount of fluid deficit may be accomplished by any of several methods:

1. Tabulation of the fluid intake and output for the preceding several days, from the history.

2. Actual measurement of weight loss over the period of a few days. Weight loss over longer periods of time will represent loss of flesh as well as water.

3. Clinical picture expressed in terms of per cent of body weight loss of fluid (p. 53).

Example Case. A 59-year-old man, given antibiotics for a sore throat, developed a diffuse stomatitis and esophagitis 5 days previously. He had taken little fluid during this time and on admission was found to have lost about 10 lbs. (originally 154 lbs. or 70 Kg.). Clinically, he presented the picture of a rather marked dehydration, which may be expressed as a loss of 6 per cent of body weight, or 4.2 L. (9.3 lbs.). This corresponds with the measured weight loss of 10 lbs. The serum NPN was 82 and the CO_2 combining power was 21 mEq./L. The urine was concentrated to 1.020 which was apparently the maximum concentrating ability.

Estimate of Requirements. The total fluid deficit has been estimated at 4.2 L. Since in water depletion this deficit is derived in proportionate amounts from extracellular and cellular fluid, the total body fluid (60 per cent) is depleted correspondingly, that is, 20 per cent from the EF and 40 per cent from the CF.

⅓ x 4.2 L. = 1.4 L., from extracellular fluid compartment.

⅔ x 4.2 L. = 2.8 L., from cellular fluid compartment.

In addition to these deficits he will require at least 2.5 L. of fluid to replace the current day's obligatory losses and to compensate for his inability to concentrate urine. Therefore, the total fluid need on the first day to re-establish water balance is 6.7 L. The sodium deficit will be at least the amount contained in the extracellular fluid loss of 1.4 L. From the cellular fluid concentration of potassium is derived the potassium deficit.

2.8 L. x 150 mEq./L. = 420 mEq., approximate potassium deficit.

Solutions Administered. Volume and osmolarity will be repaired first, and, since a metabolic acidosis exists with beginning uremia, the solution will supply excess bicarbonate rather than chloride. He is given the following:

  1,500 cc. of lactated Ringer's—to replace the EF fluid loss and the sodium contained in it at normal concentrations.
  500 cc. M/6 sodium lactate—to replace the current day's sodium need, make up sodium deficit and help correct acidosis.
  4,500 cc. 5 per cent glucose in water—to replace the remaining water deficit and the current day's requirement and augment urine volume. Of this, 500 cc. may be substituted by whole blood. To each of the last 3 L. is added 40 mEq. of potassium chloride to start replenishing the large deficit of this ion.

The order of administration should include first, a liter of Ringer's for dilution of the concentrated blood and to replace extracellular fluid volume; the unit of blood to replace blood volume and prevent hypoproteinemia; the glucose solution for increasing urinary output and treatment of uremia, and the lactate solution. The potassium should be withheld until adequate urine flow has been established (at least 300 cc. every 8 hours).

Subsequent Treatment. The volume of fluid and amount of sodium given on subsequent days will depend on the clinical condition of the patient. At least 3,000 cc. should be given daily to maintain daily balance and additional fluid may be added as indicated for the uremia. These will be in the form of glucose and water with added potassium and about 4.5

Gm. of sodium chloride for daily requirements. A multiple electrolyte solution, such as Butler's solution, may be used. If 40 mEq. of potassium were added to each of the 3 L. daily (120 mEq.) it would require more than 5 days to make up the original deficit. Thus 120 mEq. x 5 = 600 mEq. Each day, however, there will be a loss of at least 40 mEq. in the urine. Thus 40 mEq. x 5 = 200 mEq. The amount retained over loss in this period of time is 400 mEq. which is somewhat less than the original deficit. This does not take into account any extra potassium loss induced by saline infusion or loss from other sources. It has also been pointed out that in administering large amounts of potassium in intravenous solution, a considerable portion may be lost in the urine. This may amount to as much as half the quantity administered. If prolonged parenteral therapy appears likely, it is probably of advantage to administer a daily ration of magnesium. Butler's multiple electrolyte solution and several commercial preparations supply maintenance quantities of magnesium as well as phosphate.

If the dehydration has been slow in development or of long duration, a concomitant loss of blood cells and protein is likely to have occurred and the reconstruction of blood volume will leave an anemia and hypoproteinemia. The latter may cause edema which may be attributed to or confused with over-hydration from too much fluid administration. Early administration of whole blood in the marked and severe cases is advantageous, therefore.

TREATMENT OF SALT DEPLETION

The measurement of body weight does not accurately indicate the fluid loss from the extracellular fluid compartment in salt depletion since the intracellular movement of fluid which occurs in this condition will mask the actual fluid deficits. Estimation of the deficits of fluid and salt loss, therefore, may be made in the following manners:

1. Tabulation of intake and output of the previous several days from the history.

2. Clinical picture expressed as grams of salt depletion (p. 59).

3. Concentration of sodium in the blood serum (which gives only a rough approximation).

Example Case. A 60-year-old female weighing 50 Kg., was admitted for surgery. She had a blood pressure of 200/120 and had been digitalized for early cardiac decompensation. A resection for carcinoma of the descending colon was performed. Only glucose and water were given postoperatively although there was continuous gastric suction. On the fourth postoperative day the patient seemed to get worse with abdominal distention, nausea and marked weakness. On the fifth postoperative day the patient was semicomatose, had a "flaccid paralysis," and the blood pressure, which was averaging about 150/90, had dropped to 110/60. The NPN was 75. Serum sodium was 125 mEq./L., chloride 62 mEq./L. and CO_2 combining power 45 mEq./L.

Estimate of Requirements: It was decided from the clinical picture that this was a marked salt depletion representing about 35 Gm. of salt deficit. Computing this in another manner, the serum sodium level of 125 mEq./L. is 17 mEq./L. below the normal level of 142. From the total body water, 50 Kg. x 60 per cent = 30 L., one may then estimate total sodium loss:

17 mEq./L. x 30 L. = 510 mEq. deficit, (which is the amount of sodium in 30 Gm. of sodium chloride).

The difference in these two methods of estimating the sodium deficit is insignificant clinically. The hemoconcentration to some extent masks the degree of salt depletion as determined from the serum sodium level. The water deficit in this patient is approximately that amount which is lost from the EF due to drop in sodium concentration, and of this fluid loss much is due to the intracellular shift of fluid. Water deficits, therefore, are not large and will be made up partially from the overhydrated cells when sodium levels are restored. In addition, fluid to cover the current day's loss of 2,500 cc. will be required. Potassium deficiency is certain in the face of the existing metabolic alkalosis, and in a marked depletion is probably of the magnitude of 200 mEq. or more.

Solutions Administered. Osmolarity and blood volume are first repaired, and, since an alkalosis exists, excess chloride will be used over bicarbonate. It would be impracticable and dangerous to attempt to make up the sodium deficit by the use of isotonic saline since the volume required might well cause pulmonary edema in this patient with poor cardiac reserve (p. 24). Hypertonic saline will raise osmolarity with a minimum of added fluid and at the same time correct the cell overhydration. The following solutions were administered:

500 cc. whole blood—to restore blood volume, correct the shock and raise the blood pressure.

700 cc. 5 per cent sodium chloride—to supply the estimated salt deficit of 35 Gm. This is best given in two divided doses.

1,000 cc. normal saline in 5 per cent glucose will replace the existing extracellular fluid loss, dilute the hemoconcentration and supply additional chloride, as well as the current day's salt needs.

2,500 cc. glucose in water for the current day's fluid loss. To each liter, 40 mEq. of potassium chloride should be added to permit correction of the alkalosis and for the replacement of existing potassium deficits.

The order of administration requires that normal saline, the hypertonic sodium chloride and blood be given first to correct the shock and oligemia. Glucose solution is given next for excretory purposes and potassium added as the urine flow is established.

In the use of concentrated saline it is especially important that frequent review of the patient's status be undertaken and the treatment schedule be recomputed on the basis of the patient's changing condition. Intake and output charts must be kept in order that daily losses may be compensated. Moore warns that saline intravenously given at a rate faster than it is utilized will cause an increased urinary excretion of sodium. This may lead the unwary to give even larger amounts intravenously in an attempt to correct the negative balance and so overload the vascular system. If sodium levels in the urine are high with a low serum sodium then salt is being given too rapidly or there is adrenal insufficiency.

Subsequent Treatment. On subsequent days any persistent salt deficit or alteration in acid-base balance is corrected by appropriate solutions. Three liters of glucose in water with added potassium and 4.5 Gm. of salt for daily requirement should be given.

TREATMENT OF MIXED DEPLETIONS

In this, also, diminished blood volume is the primary concern of treatment after which the multiple deficiencies need to be corrected. The general principles discussed in the treatment of water depletion and salt depletion apply here as well.

Example Case. A 58-year-old, 145-lb. man was admitted with long standing anorexia, recent vomiting and loss of weight in the last week of about 12 lbs. Blood pressure was 130/90, and NPN was 92. X-ray examination showed a pyloric obstruction and, after 1 L. of normal saline intravenously, a subtotal gastric resection was done for a chronic obstructing pyloric ulcer. The day after surgery the serum chloride was 74 mEq./L., and the CO_2 combining power was 50 mEq./L. The patient showed evidence of marked dehydration of the mixed type and the blood pressure remained about 100/60. The urine output was 200 cc. in 24 hours.

Estimate of Requirements. The picture was consistent with about 8 per cent of body weight loss. In a 145-lb. man this is about 12.5 lbs. or 5.6 L. If the loss of fluid was proportionate from both fluid compartments:

$\frac{1}{3}$ x 5.6 L. = 1.8 L.—extracellular fluid loss.
$\frac{2}{3}$ x 5.6 L. = 3.8 L.—cellular fluid loss.

Since this is a mixed depletion, however, there is a proportionately greater EF loss than CF. It is therefore fair to estimate a 2.8 L. EF loss and 2.8 L. CF loss. In addition, he will require 2.5 L. for the current day's fluid losses for a total of 8.1 L. In mixed depletion the salt loss will be greater than would be indicated by 2.8 L. of isotonic saline (25 Gm.). Potassium loss may be roughly estimated as follows:

2.8 L. of CF x 150 mEq. = 420 mEq.

The alkalosis is a consequence of loss of gastric fluid and must result in even greater cellular potassium deficit.

Solutions Administered. Blood volume and osmolarity are repaired first, with the metabolic alkalosis requiring excess chloride rather than bicarbonate. Strictly speaking, hypertonic saline could be used to replace the salt deficit after rehydration has progressed to some degree. After fluid deficits have been made up, salt administration should be carefully evaluated if actual serum sodium determinations are not done, because of the danger of overhydration and cardiac decompensation. Here again frequent re-evaluation of the patient's fluid status is important. The following solutions were administered:

  2,000 cc. normal saline—for replacement of EF volume and partial salt replacement.
  500 cc. of whole blood—for reconstruction of blood volume.
  1,500 cc. of lactated Ringer's or an equivalent amount of hypertonic saline—to correct the hypo-osmolarity and remaining salt deficit.
  4,500 cc. glucose in water for cell rehydration and replacement of current day's losses. To each liter, 20 mEq. of potassium chloride may be added. Magnesium salts may also be added if indicated from the history or clinical picture.

In all patients with profound depletion the administration of fluid must be kept within the limits of the patient's ability to assimilate them. Especially in those with severe deficits and those in poor general condition, constant review of the state of hydration needs to be made. In these patients the prescribed fluid therapy can be divided into three equal portions over the 24-hour period. After each 8-hour period of therapy a review of the patient's status and degree of improvement will point up the urgency of further treatment or the lack of need for it.

The solutions given for therapy in a young and otherwise healthy individual with good cardiac reserve, when given at the same rate to an elderly individual or one with poor cardiac function, might precipitate heart failure and acute pulmonary edema. Too vigorous therapy is not necessary and may do serious harm. Once the total deficit has been estimated, replacement of only half of the total on the first day means that the patient should be 50 per cent better the next day, and the remaining solution then can be given.

Concurrent with therapy, accurate fluid and electrolyte output records must be kept to judge the degree of retention of the fluids given and to insure that losses do not keep ahead of replacement. Continuing checks of blood count or hematocrits, NPN and electrolyte determination of serum are an aid to following the course of therapy but are not absolutely essential to proper management.

CHAPTER TEN

Edema and Diuretics and Water Intoxication

The fluid imbalances so far discussed are found most commonly when a disproportion exists between the intake and output of either water or electrolytes. Edema, on the other hand, is usually a manifestation of some intrinsic defect in the normal circulation of fluids within the body, resulting in the over-expansion of the extracellular compartment (Fig. 25). The disproportion between intake and output of fluid and electrolytes is secondary to this. The defect which leads to edema may be initiated in any one of the factors instrumental in removal of fluid from the tissues as described by Starling (Chap. 2). Fluid brought to the tissues is forced across the capillary membrane by the arterial hydrostatic pressure which exceeds the pull of the colloidal protein in the plasma. Removal of the fluid from the tissues depends upon venous hydrostatic pressure, protein osmotic pressure, an intact semipermeable capillary wall, tissue tension and lymphatic flow. Although the abnormality which results from alteration in any of these factors cannot be considered a primary defect of fluid and electrolyte metabolism, ultimately the retention of water and salt produces the clinical picture of edema, as will be shown.

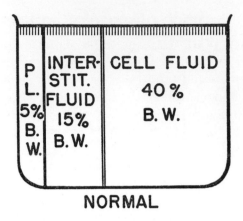

NORMAL

EDEMA

FIG. 25. Body fluid compartments and edema. The greatest increase in volume occurs in the interstitial fluid, which may retain 10 to 12 times as much fluid as the plasma. Cellular fluid may, or may not, be expanded, depending on the tonicity of the extracellular fluid and the metabolic state of the cell. Plasma volume is also increased even though it still remains the same fraction of the total body weight. Because of the expanded interstitial fluid volume, cell fluid now becomes a lesser percentage of the total body weight, while interstitial fluid is relatively greater.

DEVELOPMENT OF EDEMA

Capillary Wall. Damage to the capillary membrane or alteration in its permeability may permit the exudation of the plasma protein and fluid into the interstitial tissue. Inflammations and hypersensitivity reactions most commonly occur as localized processes, and the edema so produced is limited, therefore, to the area affected. More extensive capillary membrane changes, such as occur in generalized urticaria or other allergic reactions and in generalized sunburn, may cause considerable exudation of fluid and depletion of blood volume. The edema of acute glomerulonephritis has been attributed to diffuse capillary disease, although this explanation has been subject to criticism.

Venous Pressure. The osmotic pull of plasma protein draws water back into the capillaries as long as this force of about 22 mm. Hg exceeds the venous hydrostatic pressure of 12 mm. Hg in the recumbent position. When standing, however, the venous pressure in the column of fluid in the lower extremities rises to nearly 90 mm. Hg and an exudation of plasma tends to occur. Ordinarily, this is prevented during walking or other motion by increased lymphatic flow and by the massaging action of the muscle which reduces the venous pressure to about 30 mm. With the development of varicose veins and destruction of the venous valves the efficiency of the muscle action is lessened, and this, coupled with the capillary anoxia resulting from relative stagnation of the blood, leads to edema in these individuals. In marked obesity the venous channels embedded in the fat layers do not receive the benefit of muscular activity and edema is prone to form. Obstruction of the veins, as in thrombophlebitis or in venous compression from growths, results in a chronic increase in venous hydrostatic pressure which is slow to drop in recumbency. Tight garters produce a similar effect. The increased venous pressure of heart failure, regardless of whether it is the cause or effect of salt retention, produces edema. Edema which develops for any reason tends to accumulate in dependent regions because of the added factor of increased venous hydrostatic pressure in these areas and gravitational effects.

Plasma Proteins. Diminution of plasma protein concentration decreases the osmotic pull of fluid back into the vessels. There is no critical level below which edema will always appear, since the other factors involved in fluid shift also will play a part. Generally, however, plasma protein concentrations below 4.5 mg. per cent are associated with edema. The large losses of albumin occurring in nephrosis, amyloid kidneys and in the intercapillary glomerulosclerosis of diabetes (Kimmelstiel-Wilson's disease) produces the characteristic edema and anasarca seen in these patients. Protein loss may occur in extensive purulent infections and after repeated paracenteses for ascites. In liver disease and in hyponutritional states the low blood protein levels are conducive to edema formation. Patients with chronic dehydration treated by large amounts of intravenous solution will develop edema as a result of dilution of the blood proteins; this may be mistaken for overhydration due to too much administered saline.

Lymphatics. The edema which follows obstruction of lymph flow is said to be high in protein content. It may follow trauma involving the lymphatics and is common after the block dissection of lymph nodes for malignancy. Inadequate supporting structures for the lymphatics in the lower extremities has been suggested as a cause of the edema frequently seen in obesity. This edema may become more marked in hot weather and may be exaggerated where venous factors increase the formation of tissue fluid.

Tissue Tension. The appearance of clinical edema is earliest at sites of low tissue tension, and, therefore, first appears in loose structures such as periorbital and genital tissues. In part, the rapidity of development of pulmonary edema probably is due to the areolar structure of the lungs along with increased hydrostatic pressure in the pulmonary vein. As edema forms from any cause, the tissue pressure increases, thereby tending to stop the exudation of more fluid.

SECONDARY FLUID AND ELECTROLYTE FACTORS

In considering the above initiating causes of edema, it will be noted that in each something starts a movement of fluid out of the blood vessels into the interstitial tissue. If this were the end of it, there would result a new equilibrium in which the balance of factors in most cases would bring a halt to the continued fluid loss. Instead, the resulting drop in blood volume, as fluid moves out of the capillaries and is not returned, becomes the stimulus for adrenal mineral-corticoids which increase salt reabsorption by the kidney tubules. The resulting hypertonicity of salt concentration in the blood now stimulates the osmoreceptors in the posterior pituitary to produce antidiuretic hormone with increased water retention and increased water ingestion (thirst). As a consequence of this, several liters of edema fluid may be deposited in the extracellular compartment. With local edema, as in thrombophlebitis or in dependent edema due to venous pressure, the amount of fluid retained may be moderate, and during nocturnal recumbancy a diuresis occurs which eliminates the fluid excess retained during the day.

In the more generalized edema of nephrosis, cirrhosis and cardiac decompensation replenishment of blood volume by the salt and water does not stop the continued sodium reabsorption for some reason, and the edema may increase to tremendous proportions. Why the hypervolemia does not inhibit the adrenal hormone formation has not been explained. It has been suggested that perhaps the expansion of extracellular fluid volume does not occur at a point where it might influence volume receptors. Thus, it has been proposed that receptors may be located in the brain, and, since expansion of the interstitial fluid in the lower extremities takes place at the expense of blood volume, it is accompanied by a decreased blood flow in the head region with a continued stimulus for increasing the blood volume occurring. Experimental evidence for this effect exists in that in the sitting position, the compression of the neck veins, which congests cranial circulation, causes an increased salt excretion. In cardiac decompensation, however, neck compression does not lead to salt loss. Leaf has demonstrated the presence of an antidiuretic substance in those edematous individuals with a low sodium level, which is contrary to what might be expected in the presence of hypervolemia. However, others feel that these substances are a nonspecific result of many disease processes.

Another peculiarity of this edema is that, frequently, water is reabsorbed in proportionately greater amounts than sodium, so that blood sodium levels are apparently diluted and, therefore, are below normal—in the range of 130 to 135 mEq./L. Under ordinary conditions a dilute serum of this type should depress antidiuretic hormone production, water would be lost and the edema would be reabsorbed. The delayed water diuresis characteristic of salt depletion is also found in these edematous individuals, and the water so retained contributes to the hypo-osmolar state. Leaf and Mamby have demonstrated that the response to a water load in these individuals is identical with that produced by administration of small doses of posterior pituitary extract. These patients have a dilute serum, a concentrated urine and fail to diurese the water and dilute the urine. These investigators offer the suggestion that perhaps the stimulus for the abnormal diuretic pattern is a reduced volume in some segment of the extracellular compartment, possibly the blood volume.

OTHER CAUSES OF EDEMA

Besides the factors leading to edema, which have been discussed, any other mechanism which augments salt reabsorption by the kidney tubules may result in edema formation. This is the explanation for the edema of cortisone administration and it may also play a part in the edema which results from excessive administration of the sex hormones, such as progesterone, testosterone and estrogen. Premenstrual edema has been attributed to the salt retaining properties of progesterone and estrogen. Some drugs apparently cause salt retention, and edema is seen following the administration of the antiarthritic drug, Butazolidine. In cardiac decompensation, it is felt by many investigators that the primary step in edema formation is salt retention, rather than increased venous pressure from backup of blood as the cardiac output diminishes. In the normal individual, the standing or sitting position causes a retention of sodium, probably due to a drop in blood volume in the upper portions of the body as discussed above. Recumbancy or head-down position, on the other hand, produces a diuresis of water and salt. It has not been shown that these same changes occur in the edematous cardiac. Hemorrhage or loss of blood or serum in large quantities likewise stimulates the salt retention which here serves the useful purpose of maintaining circulating volume.

THERAPEUTIC IMPLICATIONS

Salt. Since the ultimate result in edema formation is a retention of salt, regardless of the initial cause, and with it a proportionate or greater amount of water, the usual large amounts of salt in the normal diet will contribute to an increase in edema. On the other hand, restriction of salt to the amount which is lost daily will ordinarily produce a diuresis as the retained sodium is gradually excreted. The amount permitted in the diet will be variable in different patients and will depend upon such factors as the severity of cardiac damage, renal function, amount of physical activity, nutritional state, etc. The empiric control, by trial and error, of the amount of dietary salt is probably the best clinical method of management of patients with edema, although actual measurement of daily salt loss in the urine may be of help. Dietary limitation of salt to 1 Gm. (400 mg. of sodium, or 17 mEq.), or even less, is permissible if larger amounts are not being lost by other routes, such as by the use of cation exchange resins and diuretics. It should be understood that severe salt depletion may exist in the presence of edema, and the edema may become refractory to treatment until the salt deficit is corrected (p. 135).

Water. Administration of water alone to an edematous patient will not ordinarily increase the edema unless given rapidly in large quantities. Likewise, the restriction of fluid serves no purpose since the water will be excreted unless extra salt is added to hold it. As a minimum allowance, the daily obligatory requirement of 1,500 cc. of water for evaporative loss and urinary excretion should be insured, since these patients may develop dehydration even though edema remains. Edema fluid itself is not readily used by the body for obligatory fluid requirements.

Protein. In the edema of nephrosis or other marked hypoproteinemic states, the administration of intravenous salt-poor human albumin corrects the defect and relieves the edema. The administered albumin, which is hypertonic, raises the serum protein osmotic pressure, augments the blood volume, stimulates salt excretion and results in mobilization of the edema fluid. Unfortunately, the action is only temporary in nephrosis and, as the albumin is lost through the kidneys, edema reaccumulates.

Cation Exchange Resins. These complex polymers are insoluble and nonabsorbable resins with chemical side chains having the ability to take up sodium and other cations in exchange for ammonium and hydrogen ions which they release. The compound is then eliminated through the bowel and the ammonium and hydrogen are absorbed by the intestine. The amount of sodium which may be removed both from the ingested food and from sodium present in the intestinal secretion is dependent upon the particular resin used, the amount given and the amount of sodium available in the diet. Since there are several variables in this, it is impossible to state how much sodium may be removed unless fecal sodium is actually measured. When the diet contains 9 mEq. (200 mg.) of sodium daily, an average of .3 mEq. of sodium per gram of resin is removed. Probably its main value in prolonged administration is that it reduces the number of mercurial injections required to maintain the patient in the edema-free state. To avoid the excessive loss of potassium, this cation has been substituted for some of the ammonium or hydrogen ions in various commercial preparations, which, however, reduces the efficiency in sodium removal. Since calcium may also be removed by these resins, the diet should be supplemented with additional calcium in patients to whom the resins are administered over a long period of time.

The released ammonium and hydrogen are absorbed by the intestine as the chloride. The tendency to develop chloride acidosis can be avoided by adding an anion exchange resin which removes the chloride. On the other hand, the absorbed chlorides have a diuretic effect also, acting in a manner similar to acidifying salts. Because of this chloride absorption, it is important to make certain that patients receiving the exchangers do not have renal damage with impaired ability to excrete anions. The dosage is ordinarily about 15 Gm. daily, after meals, with a diet restricted to 2 to 4 Gm. of salt. These large doses of resin are often accompanied by nausea and rectal irritation. Frequent checks of the blood chemistry should attend the use of cation exchangers to avoid the development of salt depletion, calcium loss and chloride acidosis.

Mercurial Diuretics. These substances prevent the reabsorption of sodium and chloride by the kidney tubules by inhibiting the carrier molecule mechanism, succinic dehydrogenase, which reabsorbs the sodium. Thus, mercurials oppose the effect of the adrenal hormone and clinically counteract the salt-retaining effect of ACTH and cortisone. With the increased excretion of salt a larger volume of urine is formed, the blood becomes hypertonic and fluid is withdrawn from the tissues. Since the excretion of sodium, as the chloride salt, involves the proportionately greater loss of chloride than sodium (as compared to blood levels), there may develop a hypochloremic alkalosis with resistant edema. Large amounts of potassium may also be excreted with mercurial diuresis. Possibly, this is related to, or the result of, the developing alkalosis. These drugs may be given intramuscularly or subcutaneously in 0.5 to 2 cc. doses depending upon the effect obtained in each individual. While it is best not to administer these oftener than every 3 to 4 days they have been used daily without apparent harm by some investigators. Muscle cramps in the extremities, as a result of rapid salt depletion, is not an unusual side effect and the severe agonizing cramps in the upper hypochondria characteristic of stoker's cramps is not infrequently seen following rapid diuresis from mercurials. Mercurials may also be given orally, but are less potent and reliable when given in this manner.

Acidifying Salts. The action of ammonium chloride already has been described (p. 95). In excreting the excess chloride, some sodium and other fixed base, such as potassium, is excreted also until the base conservation mechanism of the kidney is set in motion, reaching its peak about the fourth day. This drug may be given in enteric coated tablets, 9 Gm. daily in divided doses, for a period of 3 days. It is then withheld for 4 days, until ammonium production abates, after which it may again be administered. Most commonly it is used to potentiate mercurial diuretic effects, the latter being given at the end of a course of ammonium chloride. Potassium chloride may be used in a like manner where potassium deficiency exists. The chloride is then excreted bound to other cations.

Carbonic Anhydrase Inhibitor. The use of a carbonic anhydrase inhibitor (Diamox, a sulfonamide derivative) as a diuretic is a relatively new approach to the treatment of edema, and its true value has not yet been assessed.

As described above, conservation of sodium by the kidney rests in part on the exchange replacement of sodium from the glomerular filtrate for hydrogen formed in the tubules, the sodium being reabsorbed as the bicarbonate. The source of the H ion and the HCO_3 ions is from the carbonic acid formed from CO_2 and H_2O by the enzyme, carbonic anhydrase, which is present in the tubules. Blocking this enzyme with an inhibitor deprives the kidney of the H ion so that sodium cannot be spared in this fashion. Since the H ion is also part of NH_4 production, it also inhibits this means of sodium conservation. Resistance to the drug develops if it is given continuously. Doses of 0.5 Gm. or less, no more than once daily, have been used for long periods. It may be given more often with intermittent courses of therapy. Since the sodium is excreted in the urine as the bicarbonate and biphosphate which are present in the glomerular filtrate, while chloride is being reabsorbed by the tubules, a chloride acidosis tends to develop with the continued use of these drugs. Alternation of the inhibitor with mercurials or temporary cessation of the drug helps to avoid this. What effect, if any, results from inhibition of carbonic anhydrase throughout the body by this drug is not clear. Side effects are noted in the cerebral depression, drowsiness and parathesias over the body.

Urea. Administration of large amounts of urea produces a diuresis by increasing the solute load of urine, since the reabsorption of urea by the tubules is limited. The quantity of water required to excrete the load depends on the amount of the drug which is given. Doses of 20 to 60 Gm. daily may be prescribed.

Xanthines. These are mild diuretics, the mode of actions of which is not clear. It has been suggested that they may either augment glomerular blood flow and increase glomerular permeability or increase cardiac output.

The hazard in using potent diuretics along with restriction of dietary salt must be stressed. On a salt-restricted diet carefully adhered to by the patient, the daily ration of sodium which has been administered, and, therefore, retained, can be estimated. When cation exchangers are added, the maintenance of balance becomes complicated, since there is now the unknown factor of how much is being lost. If, in addition, diuretics are used, the total loss of sodium may quickly surpass the intake. Only careful observation of the patient, a knowledge of renal status and frequent determinations of serum chemistries will enable one to avoid the complications of either salt depletion and dehydration with edema or an acid-base imbalance. These complications are discussed further in the chapter on heart disease.

WATER INTOXICATION

A comparatively uncommon, but related, condition of water intoxication gains importance because of the dramatic improvement which can be produced if it is recognized and properly treated. In effect, water intoxication does exist in the edematous individual who has developed a salt depletion along with the edema, as more fully described in the next chapter and also in Chapter 6. Aside from patients with cardiac decompensation, this syndrome is most apt to be found when the surgeon has forced fluid without equivalent amounts of salt at a rate exceeding the ability of the patient to excrete. Dilution of blood sodium occurs with the result that the cells generally become overhydrated. The most commonly occurring symptoms are headache, nausea, vomiting and excessive perspiration. Later, muscle twitching, in-co-ordination, staggering gait, severe headache, stupor and convulsions occur. Cellular overhydration and edema are not manifested by the usual signs of edema indicating interstitial fluid overexpansion, and the clinical picture may result from only minor degrees of intracellular overhydration.

Characteristically here, also, as with other conditions having a low sodium level, water diuresis is delayed and the urine volume drops markedly with a low content of sodium and chloride. The conditions of water intoxication and of salt depletion apparently differ only in the rate of development. Gradual reduction of sodium concentration causes salt depletion; rapid reduction, water intoxication. Treatment is specific by stopping fluid administration and administering a concentrated salt solution, which induces a diuresis and loss of the retained fluid. Only small amounts should be given since addition of salt to an individual with too much water will result in clinical edema.

Part Two

APPLICATION TO SPECIAL CONDITIONS

CHAPTER ELEVEN

Heart Disease

Although the clinical picture of cardiac decompensation develops as a result of a diminution in cardiac output, the first clinical manifestation of this inability of the heart to match the metabolic demands of tissue is that of fluid imbalance with the development of edema. Considerable controversy still exists at present over the exact order of events leading to edema formation in decompensation, and a number of different theories have been advanced.

One group maintains that the diminished cardiac output causes a reduction in renal blood flow and smaller volume of glomerular filtrate, so that a greater percentage of the filtered sodium can be reabsorbed in the distal tubules (forward failure). Evidence has accumulated, however, which shows that diminished renal blood flow does not necessarily cause a lower sodium output in the urine. Another group feels that the early increase in venous pressure in cardiac decompensation causes transudation of fluid in accordance with the principles laid down by Starling (backward failure). Also, that the slowing of circulation through the kidney, incident to the increased venous pressure, causes sodium retention. It does not explain why the tendency to salt retention remains in these patients, even when venous pressures return to normal and when the blood volume increases with the developing edema.

EDEMA OF DECOMPENSATION

Regardless of the mechanism which eventually is shown to be the true answer, the end result is a retention of sodium and water in excess, with consequent expansion of the extracellular fluid volume. If the normal size relationship of the plasma fluid and interstitial fluid were maintained, there would be an increase of 1 L. in plasma volume for each 3 L. of interstitial fluid. If this were so, the effect would rapidly be devastating since with the collection of 15 lbs. of edema fluid, for example, the plasma would be expanded by over 2 L., which is a 60 per cent increase. Actually the ratio of retained fluid is such that 10 to 12 times as much fluid collects in the interstitial compartment as in the plasma, possibly due to dilution of plasma protein lowering its osmotic pull, and also to the increased venous pressure opposing return of fluid into the plasma. As brought out in the discussion of edema (Chap. 10), the questions arise as to why the expanded plasma volume does not inhibit adrenal hormone and, subsequently, salt reabsorption, and, also, why the hypotonic plasma does not inhibit pituitary antidiuretic hormone and, thus, diurese water. Addition of extra water to the cardiac does not produce the usual diuresis of dilute urine within 4 to 5 hours as found in the normal individual. Instead, water is retained as if in an attempt to maintain the blood volume which is already overexpanded. In the similar situation of delayed diuresis found in salt depletion and in Addison's disease, where retention serves a useful purpose, the presence of excess antidiuretic hormone has been demonstrated, but the reason for such an excess in cardiac decompensation, if it exists, is still obscure.

EFFECT OF SODIUM WITHDRAWAL AND DIURESIS

While there seems to be some disagreement as to what concentration of sodium is found in the serum in cardiac decompensation, several investigators maintain that the low serum sodium levels, which have been reported, are the result of diuretic therapy; especially of the mercurials. In a large series of patients with untreated congestive failure, the serum sodium levels were found to be appreciably above the upper levels of normal, but dropping below normal after diuretic therapy was instituted. This would more nearly conform to what might be expected if sodium retention is the first step in the formation of edema. It has been postulated by these same investigators that circulatory insufficiency alters the cellular metabolism in such a way that an osmotically inactive base (potassium) is freed from its protein-bound state, thus becoming osmotically effective and increasing the intracellular osmolarity. The homeostatic response to this in the extracellular fluid is sodium retention, raising the extracellular osmolarity to equal that which exists within the cell. The end result is edema; as recompensation occurs, the reverse process takes place, and the edema disappears.

The low serum sodium levels which are found in cardiac edema may be described under three sets of circumstances. In the presence of simple cardiac edema uncomplicated by other factors and after treatment with diuretics, the serum levels are apt to be somewhat lower than normal, although not markedly so. This may be attributed to a diluting effect by water which is retained in proportionately greater amounts than is sodium, so that levels of 132 mEq./L. or above are found. Whether this occurs as the result of too much ADH production is still a moot point. At any rate, a depressed sodium concentration is commonly found and may remain until the edema is relieved. Addition of extra salt does not raise the blood sodium level, but only adds to the edema.

A second type of hyponatremia is found in long standing edemas in which the blood levels may be lower than 130 mEq./L., and yet with no symptoms of salt depletion present. This is apparently related to the hypo-osmolar state seen in poor nutritional subjects and in pulmonary tuberculosis as described in Chapter 6 (p. 60). Those investigators who have found initially high serum sodium levels, present the idea that repeated episodes of decompensation result in excessive loss of intracellular base. Therefore, lowered cell osmolarity results, which is reflected in the extracellular fluid by a lowered sodium concentration. Apparently a new level of osmotic equilibrium has been established and addition of concentrated salt to these patients does not raise the serum sodium level, but merely increases the edema.

Restriction of salt in edematous patients is obviously a proper procedure and movement of water out of the body can be induced as sodium is slowly excreted in the absence of any salt ingestion. However, in some severe cardiacs, in spite of an overexpanded extracellular fluid volume, vigorous diuresis of sodium may lead to the third type of hyponatremia. This results in a salt depletion syndrome similar to that seen in the nonedematous individual, which is associated with a drop in blood volume, lowered cardiac output, diminished renal flow, elevated NPN and the other clinical manifestations of salt depletion. Blood levels of 120 mEq./L. or less are not uncommon. In these patients replacement of sodium in concentrated form is specific therapy with marked improvement in the clinical picture and decrease in the amount of edema. The level of sodium concentration which results from such treatment may be in the range of the hyponatremia discussed above, rather than at the normal 142 mEq./L.

EFFECTS OF FLUID WITHDRAWAL

The commonly occurring hypotonicity of edema produces, as one might expect, an overhydration of the cells. The osmotic tension in the cell becomes equal to that in the interstitial fluid both by this dilution and also by the loss of cellular electrolytes. The loss of potassium during the formation of edema has been reported by several investigators and some have found an intracellular shift of sodium. The effect of withholding water to a point below the daily loss (evaporative and urinary) leads to intracellular dehydration in the presence of edema. The plasma and edema fluid become more hypertonic with some loss of edema fluid, and the sodium concentration now may be normal or even elevated. Fluid is now withdrawn from the cell with eventual dehydration (Fig. 26). Thus the individual still shows interstitial tissue-pitting edema, but is also dehydrated, manifesting the thirst and other symptoms of this state. Additional potassium depletion of marked degree may be a result.

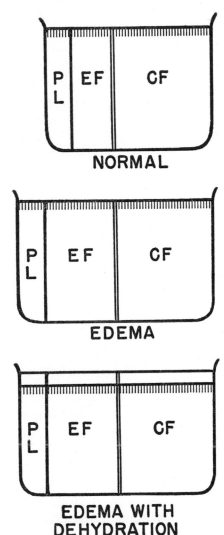

NORMAL

EDEMA

EDEMA WITH DEHYDRATION

Fig. 26. Body fluid compartments in edema with dehydration. Although the extracellular (EF) fluid is overexpanded with edema fluid, an increase in the concentration of electrolytes, because of relative water deficit, leads to removal of cell fluid (CF) with resulting cellular dehydration. Excessive loss of cellular potassium following mercurial diuresis, and inadequate food intake, will cause cell dehydration in a manner similar to that which occurs in a normal individual.

ACID-BASE CHANGES

Often in the milder forms of decompensation with moderate edema, there is found a mild acidosis, due in part to lowered sodium concentration and in part to slowing of blood circulation, thus impeding the excretion of metabolic acids and carbon dioxide. As pulmonary edema forms with interference of air exchange, blood bicarbonate increases, chloride is excreted and a respiratory acidosis results. Slowing of cerebral blood flow may also affect this by way of the respiratory center, and oxygen therapy may aggravate the acidosis, as described in Chapter 8 (p. 87). It is important that the elevated CO_2 combining power of this respiratory change not be confused with the hypochloremic alkalosis described below, since the therapy of one is not necessarily proper treatment for the other. Actual determination of the serum pH or total bicarbonate and alkali reserve are necessary for properly identifying acidosis or alkalosis. Following mercurial diuresis, which produces a relatively greater chloride loss than sodium, a metabolic alkalosis may be found, while the use of Diamox leads to selective chloride reabsorption, sodium loss and a metabolic acidosis. In severe salt depletion with diminished renal blood flow, a renal retention acidosis may result and may be added to an already upset acid-base relationship. Measurement of urinary chloride as a means of determining salt intake is obviously of little value, since, in the development of acid-base abnormalities, these ions are excreted independently of each other.

MANAGEMENT OF CARDIAC EDEMA

The primary objective in the management of congestive heart failure is improvement of cardiac efficiency, and this requires, in most cases, the use of digitalis or its derivatives along with physical rest. Restriction of salt in the diet to 1 Gm. daily (400 mg. of sodium) more or less, at least counterbalances the salt retaining tendencies in heart failure. The use of the diuretics discussed in Chapter 10 is an important means of supplementing the low salt diet and permits the more rapid removal of already accumulated excesses. The clinical management of the patient with congestive failure centers in keeping him at edema-free "dry weight," and this requires a careful balance between daily activity and salt intake. With a diet of moderate salt restriction, an increase in activity may increase sodium retention and induce more acute symptoms of failure. In a patient at strict physical rest, a meal with liberal salt intake may do the same. Anticipation of salt and water retention, as before a day of excessive activity or before a meal eaten "out," may warrant the administration of a diuretic immediately preceding or after the event. Since minimal amounts of fluid retention may be undetectable by physical findings, the daily record of weight changes may demonstrate subclinical accumulation of edema. However, this may be misleading under certain circumstances. For example, obese cardiacs carefully following reducing diets may suddenly show a decreased rate of weight loss as a manifestation of fluid retention even though the weight continues to drop. The unpalatability of the low salt diet frequently results in loss of appetite and flesh, and edema may accumulate although the weight remains stationary. In both of these circumstances, sudden onset of pulmonary edema may be the first evidence of retained fluid which has accumulated over a period of days or weeks. Administration of diuretics may then reveal a considerably lower "dry weight," as a consequence of actual weight loss. A loss of up to 2 lbs. following a mercurial diuretic can be expected even in normal individuals. This is rapidly regained, but a loss greater than this is good presumptive evidence of subclinical edema.

REFRACTORY CARDIAC EDEMA
Low Salt Syndrome

It has been pointed out that in treated congestive failure there is a tendency to retain water in spite of the fact that concentrations of sodium drop below normal, i.e., water is retained in excess of salt. Rigid restriction of salt intake, or the use of cation exchange resins, along with vigorous salt diuresis by means of mercurials or other diuretics, may cause a marked drop in concentration of sodium in the blood. This is accompanied by the signs of true sodium depletion. Likewise, while on a low salt diet the onset of vomiting, diarrhea, hot weather or other losses may bring on this condition. When this stage of salt depletion is reached, these patients no longer show the usual diuretic response and edema increases in spite of mercurial or other diuretics. Clinically, these patients appear quite ill with abdominal and muscular cramps, weakness, lethargy, anorexia, nausea and vomiting, elevation of NPN and, finally, prostration. Usually, the urine is low in volume and concentrated, if no renal damage exists, and contains minimal amounts of sodium unless the whole picture results from a salt-losing nephritis. This low salt syndrome is dramatically corrected by giving concentrated saline intravenously as in other types of salt depletion. In order to raise the blood sodium concentration, water intake must be held down to the actual daily requirement to avoid a dangerous increase in edema.

In calculating the amount of concentrated saline to give, one should theoretically base this on the total body fluid volume, including the edema fluid, as described in Chapter 9. In the presence of edema, administration of hypertonic saline intravenously may be dangerous in that it may cause a sudden expansion of blood volume and precipitate pulmonary edema. For this reason, only a fraction of the calculated amount should be given at one time. Also, as diuresis progresses, the body fluid volume diminishes so that less sodium is needed. One may avoid giving too much saline by planning to raise the sodium level to about 130 mEq., which may be near the upper limit of osmolarity in the edematous patient.

For example, take a 120 lb. patient who has gained 17.6 lbs. of edema fluid and has a blood sodium level of 120 mEq./L.

50 Kg. x 60 per cent =   30 L. normal body fluid
17.6 lbs.   =   8 L. edema fluid
The total fluid,   =   38 L., needs to be raised 10 mEq. to
                         a final level of 130 mEq./L. of
                         sodium.
38 L. x 10 mEq.   =   380 mEq. deficit.

This could be given as 450 cc. of 5 per cent saline, administered in two divided doses.

Schroeder determines the deficit by using the conservative figure of 20 per cent of the original body weight plus the volume of edema fluid as the basis for calculation. This is multiplied by the difference between the actual sodium concentration and the normal of 142 mEq. This amount will usually correct half the total deficit in 24 hours, and the remaining deficit is then recalculated. The serum sodium level may return to normal with the treatment and later drop to a hyponatremic level of a less severe degree. In some patients it has been reported that the rise in sodium concentration was preceded by a further temporary drop. It is probably of advantage to give potassium to these patients as well as to make up any calcium deficit incident to the acidosis or to the loss produced by previous mercurial diuresis.

Hypochloremic Alkalosis

The diuresis produced by mercurials is ordinarily accompanied by a tendency to metabolic alkalosis. After vigorous diuresis with mercurials, marked depression of serum chloride with elevation of CO_2 may result, and the individual loses his ability to respond to these diuretics. The symptoms of lethargy and anorexia appear as the alkalosis develops. Replacement of chloride, by giving large doses of ammonium chloride, corrects the alkalosis, and the patient again responds to mercury. Although considerable loss of potassium also occurred in the reported cases, amounting to as much as 10 per cent of the total body potassium, and although the blood levels of potassium became abnormally low, no clinical signs of potassium depletion occurred, and the electrocardiogram was normal. In Schwartz's cases, potassium was not given in treatment, but apparently the patients were eating and replacing this ion in this manner.

Dehydration and Potassium Depletion

These might be classed as refractory edemas in the sense that edema exists in dehydrated individuals in spite of deficits of cellular fluid. The occurrence of dehydration in the edematous cardiac was not infrequent in the days of treatment by the

Karell diet, and it is still a not uncommon occurrence, resulting from general debility, intercurrent infection and the nausea of digitalization. As in dehydration in noncardiac patients, this cell fluid loss will be accompanied by loss of potassium. Severe potassium loss has been reported in patients with cardiac decompensation in experiments measuring its retention during recovery. It has been shown by many investigators that a diuresis of potassium follows the administration of mercurials. It seems understandable that these patients, who are receiving diuretics, may develop severe potassium depletion, especially if there are associated nausea, diminished food intake and dehydration. There seems to be no reason why a cardiac who develops a potassium depletion from continued loss and inadequate intake should not develop the picture of hypochloremic alkalosis as described by Darrow, as well as the chloride-loss alkalosis described by Schwartz (see above). At any rate it seems worthwhile to replace potassium in these patients, orally, if possible, while diuresis is in progress, or intravenously, if necessary.

The author has seen marked diuresis induced in refractory cardiac edemas by the administration of potassium salts, despite a recent report to the contrary. This effect in the potassium depleted patient could be explained both by replenishment of deficient potassium and by the acidifying salt effect of the chloride in removing sodium in the urine (cf. ammonium chloride). Potassium chloride given in excess of that required to make up deficits, adds to the urinary solute load. This has a diuretic effect which may be advantageous.

Relation of Potassium to Digitalis Toxicity. Due to cellular potassium depletion, but apparently unrelated to serum potassium levels, the latent toxicity of digitalis may become manifest and produce the cardiac irregularities seen with overdigitalization. Replacement of potassium corrects the digitalis arrhythmia, if this was due to the potassium deficiency. It is possible, then, that dehydration or excessive diuresis with mercurials may lead to signs of digitalis toxicity, as large amounts of potassium are lost. The development of cardiac irregularities in a digitalized patient warrants the review of factors possibly leading to a deficit of the intracellular cation.

Fluid Balance in Myocardial Infarction. The amount of myocardial damage incident to an infarction may or may not be extensive enough to precipitate decompensation as the result of diminished cardiac output and anoxic damage to peripheral and pulmonary capillaries. The acute episode, however, is accompanied by the stress phenomena which have been described already (Chap. 2) and which result in salt retention and potassium excretion. The added burden of even a mild increase in blood volume may tip the scale in an infarcted heart and produce acute edema. It is logical, therefore, to restrict salt intake, at least moderately, in patients with acute infarction for a period of 4 to 5 days or until adrenal response has subsided. Edema which develops after this period is less apt to be due to stress phenomena and more to primary heart failure.

CHAPTER TWELVE

Kidney and Urologic Diseases

Upon the kidney falls the important function of adjusting the concentration of electrolytes, the extracellular fluid volume and the acid-base balance. It is for this reason that diseases of this organ, more than that of any other, are immediately reflected in derangements of the fluids and their chemical makeup. Much of the physiology involved in the formation of urine already has been discussed and a brief summarization will serve as review. The factors involved in the fluid structure of the excreted urine may be grouped under (1) glomerular filtration as influenced by (a) renal blood flow and (b) solute concentration in the blood and (2) tubular function as influenced by (a) hormonal control, (b) ion exchange and (c) excretion and reabsorption. Thus, there is a glomerulotubular balance which determines the final volume and character of the excreted urine.

Since the formation of the glomerular filtrate depends upon an adequate blood flow through the glomerulus, diminished filtration may be the result of a sudden drop in blood pressure, as in shock; dehydration, with its resultant low blood volume and increased viscosity; and, possibly, cardiac decompensation.

The rate of glomerular blood flow and its pressure are also controlled to some extent by neurogenic influences which regulate the size of the afferent and efferent glomerular arteries. Through the sympathetic nerves which control these vessels, severe emotional stimuli and pain may increase filtration pressure by constricting the efferent or dilating the afferent vessel. In crush injuries, Trueta has described a shunting of blood through the kidney medulla, bypassing the glomeruli-containing renal cortex, with a resulting anuria. The glomerular membrane does not permit the loss of protein or cells, normally, but in disease may lose both in considerable quantities. Since the glomerular urine is a protein-free plasma filtrate, the concentration of substances in the plasma will determine the concentration in the filtrate, and, this in turn, may determine the degree of reabsorption in the tubules for certain substances. For example, beyond a certain maximum blood sugar concentration the tubules cannot reabsorb all glucose and the excess is lost in the urine. This is known as the tubular maximal for that substance (Tm glucose) and such a Tm has been determined for sodium as well. One explanation for the retention of sodium in cardiac decompensation is that the diminished cardiac output leads to diminished renal blood flow, with a corresponding diminution in the glomerular filtrate. The amount of sodium presented to the tubules is, therefore, below the maximal tubular reabsorbing ability and all of the sodium is reabsorbed, with none escaping in the urine.

The tubular function of reabsorption of salt and water is an important part of the maintenance of balance. This is under the control of the posterior pituitary hormone, ADH, and the adrenal mineral-corticoids, but water reabsorption is also influenced by the solute load. Damage to the tubules in chronic nephritis results in unresponsiveness to hormonal control with loss of large quantities of water and salt. Dehydration and salt depletion may be a consequence in improperly treated nephritis. The diluting ability of the kidneys may also be impaired so that ultimately a fixed specific gravity results. In tubular damage, the inability to exchange H ion for base, and failure of NH_4 formation, leads to loss of fixed base, and this, coupled with failure of chloride and bicarbonate reabsorption, leads to acid-base imbalance. Some substances, such as potassium, are apparently excreted by the tubules as well as filtered through the glomeruli.

UREA EXCRETION

The large quantities of urea which are excreted daily give this substance an especially important role in determining the ultimate volume of urine which will be lost daily. Normally, this substance is present in the blood in concentrations of about 15 mg. per cent or, stated in other terms, 0.15 Gm. per liter. However, the urine concentration of this substance, which is in the neighborhood of 25 Gm. per liter, indicates the work performed by the kidney in this marked concentrating effort. If the amount of urea that has to be excreted daily is halved, for example, by reducing the intake of protein, the concentration of urea in the same volume of urine will likewise be half as much. The kidney will have done less work in the excretion of this load, since the concentration in the urine more nearly approaches the blood concentration. The work of the kidney in excreting urea may, therefore, be lessened also by forcing fluids, so that the load of urea can be excreted at a lesser concentration in a larger volume of urine. On the other hand, increasing protein in the diet, or decreasing fluid intake, increases the work in concentrating urea. In the diseased kidney there is a serious limitation of the concentrating capacity, and yet the daily urea load must be excreted without loss of excessive amounts of water in a dilute urine. This is accomplished by the rising blood concentration of urea resulting from inadequate glomerular filtration. For example, with the blood concentration of 15 mg. per cent, a given nephritic requires 3 L. of urine to excrete a 20-Gm. load of urea. If the blood urea is now raised to 45 mg. per cent, or 3 times its former level, the 20-Gm. load can now be excreted in 1 L. of urine, or one third its former volume, with no added work in concentrating.

Thus, elevation of the blood urea in the nephritic is the means for excreting this substance without producing a serious dehydration. Urea is nontoxic and produces no clinical effects in itself, but elevation in the blood indicates inadequate renal blood flow, and implies the retention of other materials which are poisonous. In spite of large elevations in the blood concentration of urea, it produces no fluid shifts since it easily diffuses across the cell membrane, and its osmotic effects, therefore, are equal on both sides of the membrane. This is in contrast to glucose, for example, which remains largely extracellularly and, therefore, exerts an osmotic fluid shift. Since urea does not dissociate electrically it does not contribute to disturbances in acid-base relationships.

SALT EXCRETION

The opposite state of affairs exists for sodium in respect to work performed by the kidney, since the daily load is usually excreted at a concentration in the urine which is lower than that existing in the blood. Thus, in excreting a urine with about 100 mEq./L., the tubules have had to perform work in pushing sodium back into the blood against the gradient of concentration. The work can be diminished by producing a greater sodium load so that the concentration in the urine will be the same as that in the glomerular filtrate and plasma. By decreasing water intake and urine volume the same effect is obtained and kidney work is diminished. A nephritic patient, for example, who cannot dilute urine sodium below 140 mEq./ L., may have a urine volume of 2 L., dictated by high total solute load and inability to concentrate. In this 2 L. he will lose the equivalent of about 17 Gm. of salt daily although his salt intake may be only 12 Gm. To avoid salt depletion with its consequences of lowered blood volume, diminished renal flow and further impairment of kidney function, his salt intake would need to be increased to cover his daily loss, or the fluid intake would have to be reduced to the minimum volume compatible with the excretion of the other solutes.

With the recent vogue for low salt diets in the treatment of cardiac failure, hypertension and in chronic nephritis with hypertension, many instances have been reported of salt depletion in patients unable to conserve sodium (Fig. 27). Salt loss in nephritis may, therefore, result both from failure of diluting

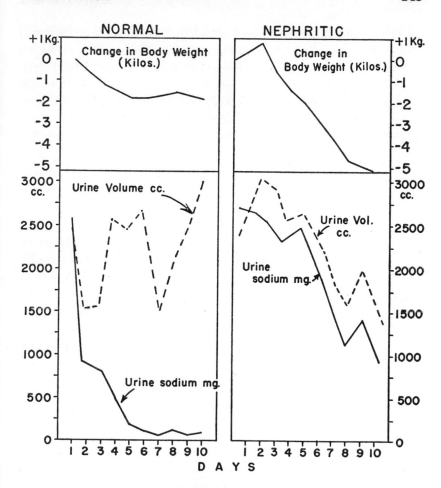

Fig. 27. Excretion of sodium in a nephritic on low sodium diet. In the normal individual, salt conservation occurs promptly and is at its maximum by the fifth day. The weight loss is moderate. In the chronic nephritic continued large sodium losses cause a marked drop in weight due to dehydration. Note the constancy of water to sodium loss due to impaired concentrating and diluting function of the tubules. (From Newburgh)

ability and from impairment of the tubular mechanism for ammonium production in the conservation of base.

In the excretion of urea and sodium it has been shown that since the work of the kidney increases as it excretes more urea, and decreases as it excretes more sodium (within certain limits), the least work for the kidney, with a normal daily solute load for these two substances, occurs when the urine volume is about 2 L.

OTHER SUBSTANCES

The excretion of potassium, which has a low serum concentration, differs from that of urea and sodium, since apparently 50 per cent of this substance appearing in the urine is excreted by the distal tubules in addition to that which is filtered through the glomeruli. As long as urine volume remains adequate, the daily load of potassium will be excreted even when glomerular filtration rate is considerably diminished. The blood level of phosphates are influenced to some degree by the blood calcium levels, with the glomerular filtration and tubular reabsorption maintaining a fairly constant concentration. Sulfates are likewise reabsorbed by the tubules to a minor extent, and diminution in glomerular filtration results in rising blood levels. Being part of the protein molecule, the load of these three substances in the urine depends on the amount of protein metabolized, whether taken as food or the result of endogenous breakdown.

RENAL ACIDOSIS

While the early results of kidney disease are disturbances in dilution and concentration, later effects involve the tubular reabsorption of wastes which disturb the acid-base equilibrium. Phosphates, sulfates and organic acids (lactic acid), being electrolytes, displace the bicarbonate ion in the blood, decrease the available base and lead to a metabolic acidosis, (Fig. 28). This imbalance is aggravated by the loss of fixed base (Na^+, Ca^{++} and K^+) as the ammonium production in the diseased tubules is diminished or lost. Figure 28 shows the increase in the acid radicals, R, and also indicates the drop in concentration of sodium and chloride incident to excessive loss in the urine. With the hyponatremia there will also be a drop in plasma volume which diminishes renal blood flow and aggravates the acidosis.

Elevation of the blood phosphate level ordinarily produces a reciprocal reduction in blood calcium by increasing calcium excretion in the urine, thus leading to parathyroid gland hypertrophy so commonly found in chronic kidney disease. Calcium is present in the serum both as ionized calcium, which influ-

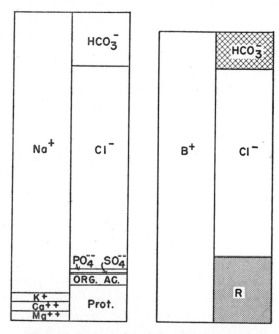

Fig. 28. Serum electrolytes in renal acidosis. (*Left*) The normal chemical structure of plasma. (*Right*) Excessive sodium loss causes a diminished total base concentration. The acid radicals, (R) are increased because of retention of SO_4^{--}, PO_4^{--} and organic acids, and the bicarbonate ion is proportionately decreased. The resulting metabolic acidosis is associated with an elevated blood urea nitrogen, which is non-electrolytic.

ences muscular irritability, and as calcium bound to protein. In the presence of acidosis, the amount of ionized calcium is increased even though the total calcium is diminished in chronic renal disease, thereby avoiding tetany. Treatment of the acidosis with alkali or sodium lactate, by reducing the ionoized calcium, may precipitate tetany unless calcium is concomitantly administered.

MANAGEMENT OF CHRONIC NEPHRITIS

Fluid Requirements. The amount of fluid administered daily will depend upon the ability of the kidney to concentrate the urine, and also upon the size of the solute load (Fig. 9). If the urine volume is maintained at 2.5 L. daily, the work of the kidney will be kept to a minimum as far as urea and salt excretion are concerned and yet permit adequate excretion of toxic metabolites. Since, under ordinary conditions, there is a daily evaporative loss of about 1,000 cc., the daily intake will have to be 3,500 cc. to permit the excretion of 2,500 cc. of urine. Other losses, such as occur in hot weather or over-exertion, will require an addition to the daily intake of the amount of the added loss. The fact that edema exists does not alter the requirements for fluid, if tubular function is impaired and there is inability to concentrate.

Diet. The solute load of urea can be controlled partially by the protein intake (80 Gm. of protein yields about 20 Gm. of urea). To maintain an adult in protein balance, about 40 Gm. of protein must be supplied daily, (0.6 Gm. per Kg. body weight). Therefore, this should be the upper limit of protein consumption. If albuminuria is also a part of the clinical picture, an additional amount of protein equal to the daily albumin loss should be added to the diet. Minimal protein catabolism is desirable, since less phosphates, sulfates and potassium are produced thereby. Endogenous protein breakdown is minimized by supplying at least 100 Gm. of glucose daily. For this reason, a diet high in carbohydrate and fat and low in protein is preferred.

Sodium. If edema is not present, there is no need to withhold sodium from the diet; it may be used as desired by the patient. If the serum sodium is found to be low, the administration of small amounts of hypertonic saline may improve greatly the condition of the patient. It is not a rare experience to find that a supposed nephritic with uremia actually has no kidney disease, and that with salt replacement for the sodium depletion, the azotemia disappears. The amount of sodium that should be administered can be judged only by the response to treatment since total losses and intracellular shifts of this ion are not measurable. On the other hand, if sodium needs to be withheld, because of severe hypertension or cardiac damage, it is important to make certain that the patient is not a "salt-loser." This can be done by placing the patient on a low salt diet for 5 days and then measuring sodium output in the urine for 24-hour periods. The quantity excreted daily represents the least amount required in the diet, plus the additional amount which must be allowed for sweat and fecal loss. In the presence of edema, salt restriction is ordinarily indicated. However, a low blood concentration of sodium may exist even in the presence of edema, when this is due to cardiac disease or to hypoproteinemia. Additional salt may aggravate the edema, and inadequate salt may worsen the renal function. The optimum compromise is to permit enough sodium to replace that which is lost.

Other Measures. The phosphate load to the kidney may be reduced by limiting its ingestion and by protein restriction. Milk contains a large amount of phosphate and so its use should be restricted. Administration of phosphate-binding substances (aluminum hydroxide gels) prevents its absorption from the intestine. Two tablespoonsful taken after meals will diminish effectively urine phosphate excretion. With milk restriction, calcium may be given in the form of calcium gluconate, 1 Gm. 3 times daily. The administration of androgens to inhibit protein catabolism and, thereby, lessen acidosis has been suggested. The anorexia and nausea which frequently occur in chronic nephritis result in insufficient food and potassium intake. This, associated with polyuria, may lead to potassium depletion unless an adequate dietary is maintained.

Intercurrent Illness. The precarious state of fluid balance in the chronic nephritic is easily upset by other illnesses. Acute diarrhea or vomiting, as a result of an ordinary enteritis, may precipitate a marked accentuation of uremia from the resulting dehydration and salt depletion. Acute illnesses in these individuals, therefore, warrant immediate hospitalization for the purpose of maintaining fluid balance by parenteral fluids.

MANAGEMENT OF RENAL SHUTDOWN

Considerable interest has been shown recently in the acute renal failure incident to transfusion reactions, crush injuries, drug poisonings and shock reactions, which are characterized by diffuse degenerative and necrotic changes in the kidney tubules. While management of renal function is of great importance, cardiac failure is probably the principle cause of death both from pulmonary edema and from hyperkalemia. Overhydration from administering too much salt and water has also been a not infrequent cause of morbidity in these patients.

PHASE OF ANURIA

Fluids. The amount of fluids given by mouth or parenterally should not exceed the daily loss, but neither should it be less. Since some water will be freed as the result of protoplasmic breakdown, the evaporative losses of 1,000 cc. need not be fully replaced. To this must be added the quantity of fluid lost as urine. Loss by vomiting, diarrhea or visible perspiration should be carefully estimated and replaced. Ordinarily, a daily intake of about 800 to 1,000 cc. of fluid is adequate if complete anuria exists.

Diet and Salt. Protein and all electrolytes should be withheld to prevent excessive retention of urea, phosphate and sulfate, and to avoid the development of hyperkalemia. Endogenous protein breakdown is minimized by administering at least 100 Gm. of glucose daily. Fruit juices, oatmeal and many other commonly used foods have a high potassium content and should be avoided. Salt deficit and shock from sodium loss by extrarenal channels may be a factor in the development of the oliguria. This ion should be replaced, using hypertonic saline if edema exists. However, if there has been no excessive salt loss it should be strictly withheld, except to replace that which may be lost by vomiting or sweat. The presence or absence of sufficient sodium is best determined by serum chemical analysis.

Dialysis. The value of the artificial kidney in acute anuria (contraindicated in acute glomerulonephritis) is still debatable. Unquestionably, normal potassium and phosphate levels and acid-base balance can be restored by its use, but the complexity of its operation makes it of limited clinical value at the present time. Peritoneal lavage is not as efficacious and carries with it some hazard of infection. Intestinal lavage is more readily available and has been reported to reduce effectively NPN and blood potassium and phosphate levels. The use of any of these procedures is warranted only in the severe anurias, since the majority of patients with acute renal shutdown will spontaneously re-establish urine flow in 7 to 15 days or longer, providing treatment has not been detrimental in the interim.

In renal shutdown with complete anuria, if intestinal lavage is contemplated, the tubes should be inserted early. This facilitates feedings in a nauseated patient, aids in relief of distention and is already in place if the need for irrigation arises. Because of the ileus and distention which is frequently present, the placing of the intestinal tubes for irrigation becomes almost impossible if delayed too long. A modification of the Miller-Abbott tube, which the author has used, may be made by removal of the bag, occluding the lumina by tying off the end of the tube and attaching a metal tip. The lumen, which is ordinarily connected to the inflatable bag, is pierced by 5 holes, spaced 1½ inches apart, about 4 feet above the suction holes, and the perfusion fluid is administered through this lumen. Suction is applied to the usual suction outlet. A typical perfusion solution consists of the following, dissolved in 1 L. of fluid:

NaCl	6.0 Gm.
NaHCO$_3$	3.0 Gm.
Calcium gluconate	0.1 Gm.
Glucose	20.0 Gm.

Irrigation is continuous at about 4 to 5 L. in 24 hours. Use of such a solution supplies glucose for caloric requirement and prevents the loss of calcium in the perfusate. Isotonicity of sodium and the presence of both chloride and bicarbonate prevent acid-base imbalance. Large amounts of potassium and nitrogenous wastes may be removed in the course of a day's treatment.

Oral cation exchange resins, without the added K^+ cycle, have been used to remove potassium with reportedly good results. The frequent presence of nausea in these patients would seem to make this procedure of limited value. Cation exchange resins given by enema have also been used for this purpose, but the amount of potassium removed in this manner is extremely variable and unpredictable. Other measures which may be used to reduce serum potassium have been discussed above (p. 72).

PHASE OF DIURESIS

If the patient improves, the oliguria is followed by a marked diuresis of water, since the injured tubules have temporarily lost their power of reabsorption. Large losses of sodium and chloride also occur which becomes a serious hazard at this stage. The fluid and electrolytes must be replaced while they are being lost in order to prevent severe dehydration or salt depletion which may develop rapidly. The total losses of fluid and electrolytes should be measured every 8 to 12 hours. The deficits between the amounts of solutions given and the losses measured should be promptly replaced. Because of the renal damage, the NPN may continue to rise in the blood even after diuresis is established and the clinical picture of uremia may become marked at this time. The vagaries of kidney function during this stage of recovery make therapy hazardous—overhydration, pulmonary edema and acidosis have been reported as causes of death after diuresis has begun. Application of the principles of management of salt depletion and acid-base balance, which have already been elaborated, are put to their severest test in the management of these patients. Laboratory determinations of blood electrolytes and losses in the urine are of tremendous help, and the use of a fluid balance service is of great advantage.

ACUTE GLOMERULONEPHRITIS

Fluid imbalance is not always a part of the clinical picture of acute glomerulonephritis, although it can become a serious problem. Opinions still are not uniform on the cause of edema, which, in the past, has been attributed to generalized capillary damage with seepage of protein into the interstitial spaces. Albuminuria with resulting hypoproteinemia is a less likely cause since edema may occur before the blood protein levels drop. Peters feels that cardiac failure and salt retention are the most likely causes of the edema, although the impaired glomerular blood flow and tubular changes play a part. The acid-base changes are not marked, unless severe oliguria results, and most commonly show an increase of chloride with hyperchloremic acidosis.

In the therapy of the acute stages with oliguria, salt and fluid intake are governed by the same considerations which were discussed under the anuric phase of acute renal shutdown. Replacement of protein likewise should be governed by the minimal requirements plus the addition of the amount of albumin lost in the urine. The use of digitalis, where cardiac function warrants this, is of value. Mercurial diuretics are of little value in acute nephritis with oliguria and, because of possible damage to already diseased tubules, should be withheld. Ammonium chloride as a diuretic is contraindicated in the presence of acidosis or uremia, since the excess chloride tends to accentuate any existing acid-base imbalance.

NEPHROTIC STAGE OF GLOMERULONEPHRITIS

The large losses of albumin decrease the protein osmotic effect of the blood and is the cause of edema in this condition. Here, again, the principles of therapy, which have already been discussed, may be applied. Salt restriction is important in nephrosis, but, since anuria is not a factor in this phase, restriction of fluid and protein is not indicated. The loss of large amounts of albumin warrants increased dietary protein, although the value of this in raising the serum albumin concentration is doubtful. By specifically correcting the protein abnormality, intravenous salt-free human albumin induces a prompt diuresis, but, unfortunately, the effects are only transitory. Urea administered orally as a diuretic has been found to be of value, but fluids must be restricted during its administration. Its action is to increase the urinary solute load and thus draw fluid with it in its excretion. Mercurial diuretics have been used for long periods with good diuresis and no apparent ill effects. The use of ACTH to produce diuresis after several days administration, or following its cessation, has no definite rationale, but it has been suggested that the hormone inhibits the production of ADH from the posterior pituitary. Some investigators have shown evidence seeming to implicate the adrenal cortex and pituitary in the causation of this syndrome.

PROSTATIC OBSTRUCTION

Long standing obstruction of the lower urinary tract raises the intravesicle pressure, and this is transmitted up the urinary tract into the collecting tubules and glomeruli. Since the rate of filtration through the glomerulus depends, in part, on the intraglomerular pressure, an increase of pressure here slows filtration and also impedes renal blood flow by the compression caused by the distended tubules. The acid-base imbalance which results is extremely variable and unpredictable, but most commonly leads to azotemia and metabolic acidosis. While in cases of short duration these changes are reversible when the obstruction is relieved, in long-standing blockage the kidney tubule damage becomes structural and permanent. Removal of acute obstruction produces a diuresis similar to that found in the diuretic phase of acute renal shutdown, and here, again, careful measurement of fluid and electrolyte loss, as well as serum chemistries, is important in proper management. In long-standing obstruction, the existing dehydration and deficits which have developed will need to be made up in addition to replacing the current losses.

URETEROCOLOSTOMY

An interesting alteration of acid-base balance has been noted in patients subjected to ureterocolostomy which produces a marked hyperchloremic acidosis. The exact mechanism of its production is not fully understood but certain factors seem to be of importance. Urine being ordinarily acid in reaction with large quantities of ammonium chloride, supplies chloride and other acid ions, in excess of base, for reabsorption from the colon. Retention of urine in the lower bowel for long periods of time promotes its reabsorption and the acidosis results. Tubular damage may also be of importance in the development of the acidosis, and it has been shown that, with normal kidneys, the absorption of acid urine from the bowel does not produce an alteration in acid-base balance. In the mangement of these patients, forcing fluids insures the frequent emptying of the bowel so that the period of absorption is short. Sodium bicarbonate is administered to combat the acidosis, but the danger of increasing the total osmolar concentration of the blood must be kept in mind. A similar series of events results after uretero-enterostomy in isolated intestinal segments. Here also the factors which contribute to development of the acidosis are the length of time the urine remains in the intestinal segment, the area of intestinal mucosa in contact with the urine and the concentration of the electrolytes in the urine. Control of these three factors will prevent the hyperchloremia.

CHAPTER THIRTEEN

Diabetic Acidosis

The development of the picture of diabetic acidosis probably demonstrates better than any other condition how an initially unrelated disease process can become a most complex problem of fluid and electrolyte imbalance. Likewise, it demonstrates clearly that blood chemical determinations of electrolytes may produce what appears to be a very distorted picture of the water balance and cellular changes of an individual, unless one understands the pathogenesis of the changes.

The initial defect, which is the inability of the body to utilize glucose, results in an increasing concentration of this substance in the blood. This produces several effects which quickly begin to upset the fluid structure. The elevation of blood sugar is reflected in an increased glucose concentration in the glomerular filtrate and the glucose level here eventually exceeds the ability of the tubules to reabsorb this substance. The kidneys, therefore, are presented with an increased solute load requiring the loss of extra fluid with the resulting polyuria. The higher the blood sugar level, the more fluid will be lost in this manner. This diuresis of glucose inhibits reabsorption of sodium also, and, to a certain extent, excessive sodium will be washed out with the glycosuria. As long as the patient is mentally clear and able to help and feed himself, the polydypsia and increased intake of food and sodium will balance the excessive losses of these substances.

The second effect of the elevated blood sugar is a consequence of the essentially extracellular position of glucose as such, prior to its phosphorilation, so that the extracellular fluid becomes increasingly hypertonic with the glucose. As usual, this hypertonicity is the osmotic force leading to a withdrawal of fluid out of the cells, carrying with it the cell cations, potassium and magnesium, and the anion, phosphate. This migration of fluid into the extracellular fluid, by its diluting effect on the blood constituents, makes the true state of dehydration, as measured by the hematocrit, less apparent. In addition, the acidotic diabetic, by virtue of the lack of insulin, is in a fasting state that contributes its effect to the total imbalance, by adding cell protein breakdown with added nitrogen and potassium loss over that which is lost in the dehydration.

The acid-base distortion stems from the fact that failure to metabolize glucose leads to increased fat utilization for energy requirements, and ketonic acids, which are, therefore, produced in excess, begin to accumulate in the blood. These increase at the expense of the bicarbonate ion, leading to the development of ketosis and metabolic acidosis. In the renal excretion of ketones, which are strong acids, they are combined with fixed base, and thus aggravate an already developing sodium depletion. The additional solute load of ketone excretion results in an even greater loss of water in the formation of the acetonuria. The nausea and vomiting of acidosis, as well as the gastric dilatation frequently found in diabetic coma, also contributes to the total fluid and electrolyte loss.

The picture so far presented is due directly to the metabolic fault of diabetes, but the marked dehydration with depletion of blood volume now produces a secondary effect on renal function. With the increasing dehydration and hemoconcentration and consequent drop in blood pressure, the renal blood flow becomes inadequate, and to the already existing acidosis is added the retention of the organic acid wastes, sulfates and phosphates. Interference with glomerular filtration, as renal blood flow is decreased, also diminishes the excretion of potassium, large amounts of which are being freed into the blood from cellular dehydration and starvation. Blood levels of potassium, phosphate, sulfate and organic acids, therefore, usually are elevated.

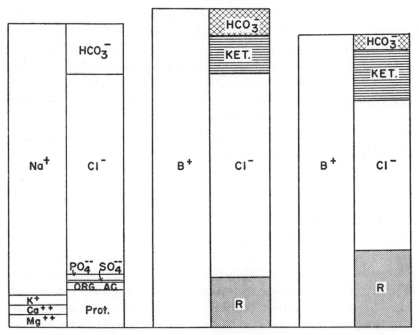

FIG. 29. Serum electrolytes in diabetic acidosis. (*Left*) The normal electrolyte pattern. (*Center*) Ketones increase at the expense of bicarbonate ions. The total osmolar concentration is increased because of dehydration, and the serum levels of electrolytes are elevated. (*Right*) Increase in the amount of ketones and in retained urinary excretory products (R) causes a marked decrease in alkali reserve. The continued sodium loss results in a low sodium concentration and a marked metabolic acidosis.

CLINICAL AND LABORATORY PICTURE

The end result, as far as volume and concentration are concerned, is a marked intracellular and extracellular fluid depletion which is clinically manifested by the well-known signs of dry mucous membranes, sunken eyes, soft eyeballs and a highly concentrated urine. Blood levels of sugar and potassium are elevated and the hematocrit is increased while the blood volume is diminished (Fig. 29). The large losses of sodium which are attributable to the dehydration, glucose diuresis, vomiting and excretion of highly ionized anions, eventually lead to a lowered serum concentration in spite of hemoconcentration. The acid-base picture is that of a severe ketosis and acidosis with a serum pH reaching levels as low as 6.9. The carbonic acid to bicarbonate ratio is upset both by sodium loss and by replacement of bicarbonate with ketones. The Kussmaul breathing of acidosis is the respiratory mechanism for excreting the relative excess of CO_2. If shock becomes a factor because of drop in blood volume, interference with the respiratory center may dangerously depress respiratory function with aggravation of the acidosis.

PHOSPHORUS AND MAGNESIUM

It is not possible at the present time to state what, if any, pathologic physiology results from deficits of these two electrolytes, but it has been reported that patients seem to improve more rapidly where these are given in treatment. In view of the marked cellular dehydration that occurs in diabetes, loss of both of these primarily cellular constituents would be expected and has been demonstrated in the amounts retained during recovery from acidosis. Their behavior follows, very much, that of potassium, so that blood concentrations of phosphorus and magnesium are increased with the dehydration and its attendant impairment of renal function, and with rehydration following treatment the blood levels fall as urine flow is established and the elements re-enter the cell. Recent evidence indicates that hypomagnesemia may be more common than formerly thought, leading to muscular hyperirritability and delirium (p. 74).

TREATMENT OF DIABETIC ACIDOSIS

Estimation of Deficit

The stage of development to which the dehydration has progressed, of course, will determine the clinical picture and indicate the quantitative requirement of replacement solutions. As has been indicated, because of the coexistance of sodium and chloride loss, hemoconcentration and partial redilution of the blood by cell fluid, the exact extent of water and salt depletion hardly can be computed from determinations of blood chemistry. This applies as well to the other electrolytes. Fluid deficiency in amounts up to 10 per cent of body weight have been shown to occur in severe acidosis. In *severe* diabetic acidosis the total deficits that may develop in a 70 Kg. individual have been computed. From the data published by Butler, they are: water, 7,000 cc.; sodium, 525 mEq.; chloride, 440 mEq.; potassium, 420 mEq.; phosphorus, 260 mEq.; magnesium, 56 mEq. In less severe dehydration these total losses may be correspondingly less.

It is of paramount importance to replace as early and as completely as possible the deficits of sodium and water, to produce a more adequate blood volume and to enhance renal function. In the first 24 hours of treatment 80 per cent of the total deficit of water and salt should be replaced. There is less urgency for the other electrolytes since the rate of assimilation of the intracellular electrolytes is limited and only 50 per cent of potassium and magnesium and 25 per cent of phosphate need to be given the first day. Therefore, replacement in the first 24 hours based on these percentages should be:

	Per Kg. Body Weight	
Water	80	cc.
Sodium	6	mEq.
Chloride	5	mEq.
Potassium	3	mEq.
Magnesium	0.4	mEq.
Phosphorus	1	mEq.

In addition to these deficits, the daily maintenance requirement must be given to replace obligatory loss of fluid along with sodium and potassium. This additional amount will need to be included daily as long as parenteral solutions are given.

In general, the therapy is guided by the same principles which were discussed in the treatment of mixed depletions in Chapter 9. Most important is adequate amounts of insulin to utilize sugars and control ketogenesis, after which the immediate requirements are to re-establish blood volume and repair extracellular and intracellular dehydration. Considerable controversy still exists over whether glucose solution should, or should not, be given early in the treatment of diabetic acidosis: equally good results are reported from both camps. It would seem that a fair compromise would be to give little or only small amounts of glucose early (first 2 to 4 hours), to avoid adding to the already elevated blood sugar level, which furthers dehydration and polyuria. As the blood sugar concentration diminishes, glucose solution should be supplied more liberally to avoid hypoglycemia and to make available more salt-free water for urine formation and other obligatory requirements. It has been pointed out by several investigators that a 2.5 per cent solution of fructose in hypotonic saline makes an isotonic solution which is probably of greater value than glucose in the treatment of diabetic acidosis. Fructose is rapidly metabolized, bypassing the site of action of insulin, and, therefore, it decreases ketogenesis and avoids the cell dehydrating effect of glucose. Only a small proportion of the ingested fructose is excreted in the urine, and the osmotic diuresis which glucose produces does not occur with this carbohydrate.

If an isotonic solution such as normal saline or 5 per cent glucose is used, dilution of the concentrated blood will occur, but free fluid then is not available immediately to rehydrate the cells and establish urine flow. It has been suggested, therefore, that in the early periods of treatment a hypotonic solution of sodium or glucose be used. In the administration of sodium, about one third of the total amount should be given as the lactate rather than the chloride, since this will facilitate the correction of the acidosis. The excess of chloride over sodium present in sodium chloride will diminish further an already dangerously low bicarbonate level. Since M/6 sodium lactate is slightly hypertonic, however, it may impede cellular rehydration and, therefore, should be diluted with other solutions so that the concentration of sodium is less than that in plasma. After the patient improves, with evidence of more adequate circulatory status and increase in urine flow, solutions containing potassium may be substituted to prevent hypokalemia and to begin replacement of existing deficits. The intravenous administration of potassium is dangerous, however, and should be avoided early in therapy while blood levels of this electrolyte are high. The use of the multiple electrolyte solution described by Butler (Table 4) or other similar solutions are of advantage in supplying magnesium and phosphate as well as potassium and lactate at this stage of the treatment.

The correction of hemoconcentration can be followed by repeated hematocrit determinations. Persistence of shocklike symptoms and failure of the hematocrit to return to normal may indicate a continued loss of fluid through the injured vascular tree. Transfusions of whole blood therefore are indicated to replace blood volume and correct shock.

Care must be exercised in administering large volumes of fluid, and the status of cardiac reserve and renal function should be considered carefully. If enough repair of deficit can be accomplished so that nausea and vomiting abate and food and liquid can be taken by mouth, this route of therapy is the one of choice, and the remaining deficits can be corrected in this manner.

Making use of the most readily available solutions, the intravenous therapy for a 70 Kg. individual in severe diabetic acidosis might be as follows:

2,000 cc. of a mixture of 750 cc. of lactated Ringer's solution
    and 250 cc. of distilled water given at 200 drops per min-

ute. This contains in each liter 96 mEq. of sodium, 84 mEq. of chloride, 24 mEq. of bicarbonate and negligible amounts of potassium.

4,000 cc. of Butler's multiple electrolyte solution at 80 drops per minute. This completes the estimated deficit of sodium and chloride and gives 92 mEq. of potassium, and 20 mEq. of magnesium in all. Glucose or fructose may be added from sterile ampules, 25 Gm. to the liter, so that the resulting solution is hypotonic.

1,000 cc. of 5 per cent glucose in distilled water with 80 mEq. of potassium chloride given at 70 drops per minute, completes the water requirement and gives a good start towards potassium replacement.

If additional lactate is desired, M/6 sodium lactate may be administered diluted half-and-half with 5 per cent glucose solution in place of the third liter of solution listed above.

In smaller individuals, and in those with less severe degrees of dehydration, correspondingly smaller amounts of fluid and electrolyte, of course, would be necessary.

DEVELOPMENT OF HYPOKALEMIA

The cellular depletion of this electrolyte may be quite marked, as shown by studies which measure the amount retained by patients under treatment, and may amount to as much as 500 mEq. in severe dehydration. Not all of this is immediately replaceable, however, since only that part lost by release of cell water can be returned with rehydration. The portion lost as part of protein breakdown will be replaced only as cell metabolism and growth takes place. In the course of therapy, the administration of large volumes of fluid with sodium and insulin corrects the ketosis and repairs the volume deficit but may produce more serious disturbance of the blood electrolyte. As dilution of the extracellular fluid occurs, the hemoconcentration is relieved, urine flow becomes more copious and replacement of cell fluid is initiated. Each of these factors has the effect of depressing the blood potassium level, in addition to which, the saline infusion washes out more potassium from the cell.

All of these taking place at once leads to a sudden marked hypokalemia, often reaching levels of less than 2 mEq./L. The patient develops shallow respirations with respiratory paralysis, electrocardiographic changes, a weak, rapid pulse and ashen color due to cardiac failure and, finally, death. Previously unexplained, these sudden deaths are apt to occur unexpectedly at a time when the patient seems to be improving dramatically; most have occurred from 8 to 20 hours after the onset of treatment. This hazard of hypokalemia can be avoided by the judicious use of potassium in the replacement solutions after rehydration is under way. Although the total body deficit cannot be made up in the first day, the immediate risk of blood potassium level depression is avoided.

Hypopotassemia with electrocardiographic change has also been reported in diabetic acidosis prior to therapy, and in this situation an even greater danger exists. Serum potassium determinations, or at least an electrocardiogram, would be of value prior to the initiation of treatment in any acidotic diabetic.

CHAPTER FOURTEEN

Pediatric Fluid Balance

The principles of fluid balance which have been presented apply equally as well to the infant, with the exception that there is less margin for error in the maintenance and treatment of the pediatric subject. This is so because the relatively greater volume of fluid exchange in infants as compared to total body water may lead to more rapid dehydration under conditions of deprivation. In Figure 30 it is seen that the normal daily intake of fluid in the adult amounts to about one seventh of the total extracellular fluid volume, while in the infant a volume equal to one half the extracellular fluid is replaced daily. The total water turnover in the infant is, therefore, 3 to 4 times as rapid as in the adult, making it obvious that the infant can become much more rapidly depleted than the adult. The reason for this apparent disparity in water requirement lies in the fact that the solute load in water excreted both by perspiration and urine depends on the rate of metabolism which is related to the surface area of the body rather than to the body weight. Thus an adult who weighs 70 Kg. is 10 times the weight of an infant of 7 Kg. but has only about 4 times the surface area (1.75 sq. M. as compared to 0.4 sq. M.). The smaller the individual, therefore, the greater will be the water exchange per kilogram of body weight. For the same reason, the urinary solute load based on area of body surface will be comparatively greater in the child than in the adult, so that the obligatory urine loss, with good kidney function, is 100 cc. daily in the infant as compared to the adult's 600 cc.

NEWBORN

At the time of birth the total body fluid is somewhat greater than in the adult, amounting to about 70 per cent of body weight, with the major part of the difference occurring in the EF compartment. This excess fluid is lost by invisible perspiration fairly rapidly over a period of about 3 or 4 days. After this interval the volume of urine flow increases to its usual level of about 200 cc. daily as the evaporative loss decreases. During this period of physiologic dehydration, the serum protein becomes elevated as does the hematocrit, but by the fifth or sixth day these are again within normal limits.

In the newborn, and especially in the premature infant, the ability to concentrate urine is not developed, possibly due to failure of response to ADH, and likewise glomerular clearance rates for sodium and urea are not equal to the adult. Clinically, this means that added sodium is more slowly excreted by the glomeruli. Hence, the marked tendency for infants to develop edema. On an increased protein diet, blood urea levels may rapidly become elevated. The inability to concentrate urine in the first few months indicates that under conditions of water deprivation the infant is less able to conserve water, and dehydration, therefore, develops at a more rapid rate. The renal function of regulating acid-base balance is also less efficient in the infant. The greatly increased phosphate reabsorption by the tubules, coupled with an incompletely developed mechanism for ammonium production, limits the base-conserving ability of the kidney. By simply changing the diet to one in which there are increased amounts of fixed acids to be excreted, an acidosis may be produced.

The electrolyte patterns of newborns show an increased total base which reaches adult levels in a matter of hours. Chlorides likewise are increased and rapidly drop to normal adult ranges. Carbon dioxide combining power tends to be lower, and the acidosis, which is ordinarily found, appears to be due to an increase in organic acids resulting from an anaerobic type of metabolism which occurs in the immediate postbirth period.

INFANTILE DIARRHEA

While the losses of fluid and electrolyte occasion the same types of depletion and acid-base changes seen in the adult, special significance attaches to infantile diarrhea because the changes which occur in this condition parallel those of diabetic acidosis in their severity.

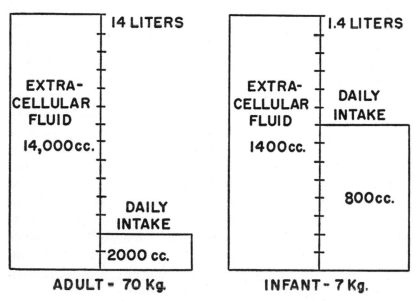

FIG. 30. Comparison of normal daily fluid intake to size of extracellular fluid compartment in an adult and in an infant. The daily fluid turnover represents about one seventh of the extracellular fluid in the adult, but about one half the extracellular fluid in the infant. For this reason, dehydration with circulatory and renal failure occurs much more rapidly in the infant. (Redrawn from Gamble)

The blood chemical picture resulting from severe diarrhea is a variable one depending on all the factors of control, such as the degree of dehydration and its effect on renal function, amount of vomiting, perspiration and the ability of the child to retain food. The rate of water loss exceeds that of electrolytes in hot weather so that a hypertonic dehydration results, but, without the added factor of excessive perspiration, electrolyte loss exceeds the fluid and a hypotonic dehydration occurs instead. Blood volume becomes depleted and may progress to the point of shock with cold, pale extremities and markedly diminished renal flow, with resulting acidosis. Cellular depletion also occurs, both as a result of dehydration and of starvation, so that large deficits of potassium, magnesium and phosphate result. The high content of potassium in diarrheic stools contributes to the great wastage of this ion. For purposes of classification the dehydration occurring in infantile diarrhea would best be termed a mixed depletion of severe degree. If the progression of the picture is rapid enough the physical findings of dehydration with loss of skin turgor may not be evident.

The losses of sodium and chloride in diarrhea, as determined by the amount retained during treatment, indicates that the total losses of these two electrolytes are apparently in the proportion normally found in serum. Darrow has demonstrated large deficits of potassium in diarrhea with the result that the extracellular sodium, already depleted, shifts into the cell, leaving a relative excess of chloride and a metabolic acidosis. This intracellular shift probably also contributes to the serum hypotonicity which is often found. The acidosis may likewise be furthered by failure of renal function incident to dehydration, and by the ketosis which results from inadequate food intake. Hyperpneic breathing is the clinical manifestation of the acidosis.

Because of the small margin which exists between the extracellular fluid volume and the daily fluid turnover a deficit of fluid intake or excessive fluid loss may cause rapid contraction of blood volume with shock and sudden death. To explain the sudden and unexpected deaths which are seen in infants with severe diarrhea, the idea has been advanced that with the progressive potassium loss a sudden shift of sodium into the cell from an already contracted plasma volume causes further loss of extracellular fluid and medical shock.

THERAPY

The magnitude of the deficits which occur in infantile diarrhea have been determined by Butler as follows:

	PER KG. OF BODY WEIGHT
Water	125.0 cc.
Sodium	9.5 mEq.
Chloride	9.0 mEq.
Potassium	10.0 mEq.

These figures represent the deficiencies which need to be made up. In addition, the daily maintenance must be added. Gamble has stated that if one fourth of the usual daily water intake and two thirds of the usual caloric intake are retained, the infant may remain in fluid balance by the adjustments in the renal concentrating mechanism, and additional parenteral treatment need not be given.

In the active therapy, Darrow stresses the fact that food by mouth should be withheld until vomiting ceases, to prevent aggravation of both the vomiting and the diarrhea, thereby adding to the electrolyte and fluid loss. During this period intravenous solutions should be given containing glucose, sodium chloride and potassium to replace the accumulated deficits as shown above, and to supply the needs for the current day. From 200 to 250 cc. of fluid per Kg. of body weight may be given parenterally in the first day to supply deficits and current needs. After this an electrolyte solution (such as "K lactate" or Butler's multiple electrolyte solution) may be given orally, and sugar may be added for caloric needs and to make the mixture more palatable. When oral feedings can be retained, this is the preferable route and Darrow recommends giving daily doses of 150 cc. per Kg. of body weight to maintain nutrition and electrolytes during the period of fasting which may last from 2 to 5 days. Following this, if food can be taken, it may be increased gradually. Again, it is important not to aggravate fluid and electrolyte loss by pushing milk, if it cannot be taken.

If shock is present, rapid replacement of blood volume is imperative. This is accomplished to some extent by the intravenous sodium chloride, but transfusions in large quantities are also of great importance (20 to 30 cc. per Kg.). The acid-base balance ordinarily needs no special therapy and will correct itself if adequate fluid and electrolyte are provided. Where the sole treatment of these cases is glucose and saline, all elements are eventually restored except the potassium, and the acidosis is converted into an alkalosis because of the potassium depletion.

A word of caution on the use of glucose in water by hypodermoclysis is added here, because of the frequent use of this route of administration in children. The severe salt depletion and EF contraction that occurs has been pointed out. This may be dangerously aggravated by the salt removing effects of electrolyte-free solutions given in the muscle or under the skin (p. 105).

CHAPTER FIFTEEN

Burns, Cirrhotic Ascites, Toxemia of Pregnancy

BURNS

While comparatively small amounts of fluid actually may be lost from the confines of the body, the depletion of fluid which results from burns may be of huge proportions. The amount of fluid exuding from the surface of a burn depends on the depth of the burn and the formation of an eschar, but the extravasation of fluid from the vascular compartment into the interstitial tissue in and around the damaged area is usually of considerable volume. The magnitude of this fluid displacement is proportional to the area of body surface involved by the burn and, to a lesser extent, the depth. This is influenced also by the presence of infection, operative procedures, anemia and by excessive fluid therapy, all of which may augment the loss of fluid into the injured tissue. The exudation occurs most rapidly in the first 8 hours following the burn and then gradually slows, reaching its maximum volume in about 36 to 48 hours. Following this, a reabsorption or relocation of the dislodged fluid occurs which may be quite rapid, but usually requires about 2 weeks for completion; even longer in the deeper burns.

173

The hemoconcentration resulting from the localized extravasation causes fluid to be drawn into the blood compartment from all normal tissues over the body so that there is a generalized dehydration for the benefit of the edema at the site of injury. The exact degree of hemoconcentration is obscured to some extent by red cell destruction at the burn site amounting in some cases to 7 to 10 per cent of the total red cell mass. The marked contraction of blood volume produces a diminished renal flow with drop in urine volume and salt retention, with this effect being enhanced through adrenal stimulation resulting from the trauma. While it has been difficult to determine the exact transfers of electrolytes which occur in the edema fluid, some evidence seems to show a shift of sodium into the burned area along with large losses of potassium from the damaged cells. If this is true, then one might expect that in the normal tissues the reverse occurs so that there is a general sodium depletion in the body as this electrolyte moves into the burn. The drop in sodium concentration results in cellular overhydration generally, which aggravates the already marked depletion of extracellular fluid volume in the body. The application of pressure dressings at the site of the burn does not influence the amount of fluid lost but merely displaces it to the surrounding tissues and may do harm in shutting off circulation to the damaged parts.

ESTIMATION OF DEFICIT

The quantitative determination of the amount of fluid to be replaced is at best a rough estimate, but can most nearly be approximated when based on the percentage of body surfaces involved by third degree burn or, to a lesser extent, by second degree burn. The "rules of nine" suggested by Wallace gives a simple method of estimating the percentage of body surface involved, by breaking up the total body surface into areas of 9 per cent or its multiples:

Head   =   9 per cent of body surface
Each upper extremity =   9 per cent of body surface
Each lower extremity = 18 per cent of body surface

Front of body   = 18 per cent of body surface
Back of body   = 18 per cent of body surface

Burns covering 20 per cent of the body surface will usually do well regardless of adequacy of fluid therapy, while those with over 50 per cent of body surface involved have a high rate of mortality in spite of careful and proper therapy. The group of burns involving 20 to 40 per cent of the body surface require careful supervision, and it is in this group that proper replacement therapy may play a life or death role. The clinical picture of dehydration with drop in blood volume is manifested by marked thirst, restlessness, hypotension, oliguria, nausea and vomiting.

Various formulae have been devised to serve as a basis for initiating therapy. Regardless of which formula is used, continued observation of the patient is necessary with review of the estimated requirements as time progresses, in order to avoid overhydration and to recognize insufficient therapy. Evans has suggested as the total fluid replacement for the first 24 hours:

2 cc. per Kg. body weight $\times$ per cent of body surface burned.

The total volume administered is divided equally between an isotonic electrolyte solution and a colloid solution (plasma or plasma expander). Where the burn covers more than 35 per cent of the body surface, the proportion should be 2 parts of plasma solution to 1 part of electrolyte solution. In addition, 2,000 cc. of glucose in water is added for the obligatory fluid loss of urine and evaporation. Thus, in a 70 Kg. patient with a 30 per cent of body surface burn, for the first 24 hours:

2 cc. $\times$ 70 Kg. $\times$ 30 per cent burn = 4,200 cc. fluid replacement

2,100 cc. as plasma
2,100 cc. as saline or lactated Ringer's
2,000 cc. of glucose and water for obligatory
needs

Total fluid = 6,200 cc.

This formula works well in patients with burns covering up to 50 per cent of the body surface (e.g., in a 70 Kg. patient, replacement and obligatory fluids total 9,000 cc.). Beyond this volume, the hazard of overloading the circulation and inducing pulmonary edema is great. (Pulmonary edema also may occur, however, as the result of alveolar damage from smoke and fumes).

Of the total volume to be given in the first 24 hours, one half is given in the first 8 hours, and the remainder is administered equally over the next 16 hours. In this way the administration of solution keeps pace with the rate of fluid extravasation into the area of burn. In the second 24 hour period, one half to two thirds of the above total volume may be given, but during the 36th to 48th hour one must watch for the diuresis that begins as the edema is re-absorbed. The quantity of fluid administered then needs only to make up ordinary daily needs (1,500 to 2,000 cc.).

The formula suggested by Cope and Moore gives similar but somewhat larger amounts. In a 70 Kg. individual with 30 per cent burn they advise for the first 48 hours:

> A volume equal to 10 per cent of body weight 7,000 cc.
> 1,000 cc. for each 30 per cent area of burn . . . 1,000 cc.
> Total fluid . . . . 8,000 cc.
> Two thirds of this is given as plasma expander or colloid and one third as electrolyte solution.

Of this total fluid, three fourths is given in the first 24 hours (one half of this in the first 8 hours and one half in the next 16 hours) and one fourth of the total is given in the second 24 hours.

> 1,500 cc. is added in each 24 hours for renal requirements. This quantity is divided into one half glucose in saline solution and one half glucose in water.
> 1,500 cc. is added in each 24 hours as glucose in water for invisible perspiration.

Thus, in the first 24 hours a total of 9,000 cc. of solution, and in the second 24 hours 5,000 cc. would be given. Oral therapy for the replacement of electrolyte and fluid, if the patient is able to take fluids, is to be preferred over the parenteral route, where this is best administered as a solution composed of two thirds sodium chloride and one third sodium bicarbonate in the required volume.

STAGE OF DIURESIS

After the first 36 to 48 hours, edema reabsorption begins and the diuresis which occurs at this stage may be very rapid and copious. Recent work has suggested that the volume of urine lost in this stage may be lessened by giving smaller amounts of fluid in the first stage. That is, the copious diuresis is partially induced by too much fluid given early in the treatment. If diuresis does not occur by the 48th hour after the burn, the suspicion of a lower nephron nephrosis must be entertained, although this is apparently rare. It has been pointed out also that a low urine output, while adequate fluids are being administered, may be the result of gastric dilatation with accumulation of fluid in the distended stomach.

Cope and Moore have found the measurement of hourly urine flow an important index of adequacy of therapy, and recommend that all severely burned patients have an indwelling catheter to measure the urine volume. The optimal rate of urine flow is between 30 to 50 cc. per hour. The appearance of less urine than this in any hourly sample indicates the need for more rapid fluid administration, while urine flow of over 100 cc. per hour indicates too much fluid. The normal rate of urine formation varies with age as shown in Table 5. If, with lower levels of urine output, doubt exists as to the presence of a lower nephron nephrosis, they suggest the following fluid test: 1,500 cc. of glucose and water or saline is given in 40 to 60 minutes. If there is increased urine flow, kidney function is presumed to be adequate and more rapid fluid administration is indicated. Failure to increase the rate of urine formation, however, indicates severe kidney damage. The possibility of gastric dilatation must be considered, and if gastric suction is required, this additional fluid loss will need replacement.

TABLE 5. NORMAL RATES OF URINE FLOW AT DIFFERENT AGE PERIODS.

AGE	URINE CC./HR.
B - 1 yr.	8-20
1 - 5	20-25
5 - 10	25-30
10 - 14	30-50
14 and older	50-100

(From Wallace)

Use of whole blood in burn cases has produced much discussion. Since hemoconcentration with elevation of the hematocrit is a paramount feature of severe burns, the addition of red cells may, with continued plasma loss into the burn area, cause an even greater red cell concentration. With a hematocrit over 60, whole blood should not be used until adequate electrolyte solution has reduced the cell concentration. The use of ACTH or cortisone in the treatment of severe burns has not gained general acceptance and there seems much, theoretically, to contraindicate their use. The losses of potassium following burns are usually of a large order and replacement of this electrolyte in the intravenous solution and orally, when tolerated, speeds the protein buildup and the replacement of the deficit.

CIRRHOTIC ASCITES

In spite of the current interest among investigators in the mechanism of formation of ascites in cirrhosis of the liver, the answer still remains obscure. It has been demonstrated that in these patients the excretion of sodium in the urine becomes minimal in spite of adequate salt intake. This diminution in salt (and water) excretion becomes evident in the early stages of liver damage and in infectious hepatitis before any fibrotic changes have occurred in the liver. Increased tubular reabsorption of sodium has been demonstrated in these patients, also, and would seem to point to some abnormality in the adrenal control of this function. This is especially so in view of the fact that the sodium retention appears to be generalized with diminished output in sweat and in saliva as well as in the urine. The not uncommon finding of a serum concentration of about 130 mEq./L. however, indicates that sodium retention may not be the primary factor in formation of ascites, since water is being retained in excess of sodium. This should implicate some water retaining or antidiuretic substance. Such substances have been identified in the urine and serum of patients with severe liver disease, as in other conditions they have been characterized by low serum sodium levels. These could result from an overproduction of pituitary ADH, from failure of the liver to destroy normal amounts of ADH or from some unknown antidiuretic substance formed by the damaged liver itself. Again the question arises as in other edemas: Is the antidiuresis primarily responsible for the ascites, or are these hormones a secondary phenomena, the result, rather than the cause, of edema?

FORMATION OF ASCITES

The actual formation of ascites is apparently controlled by the same laws which govern the movement of fluids elsewhere in the body. Cirrhotic obstruction of the portal circulation may increase the portal venous tension from about 100 mm. of water to 300 mm. or more, and yet obstruction of the portal system, in itself, is not enough to cause ascites. If liver damage is produced in conjunction with the portal obstruction, then ascites does form. The lymphatic flow becomes markedly increased when the portal veins are experimentally occluded; this along with collateral circulation, helps to remove a large part of the increased portal load. The hypoproteinemia often found in association with severe liver disease must add its osmotic forces to the exudation of the fluid. As mentioned above, the damaged liver cells, by either producing or failing to inactivate an antidiuretic hormone, decrease urine volume, increase blood volume and, thereby, increase the availability of fluid for ascites formation. The delayed water diuresis seen in other edematous low salt states is also found in variable degree in these patients, and those with the most prolonged interval before diuresis usually have the lowest sodium levels.

Administration of a water load of 1,500 cc. in the normal individual results in an excretion of 50 per cent of the load in
100 minutes. In the presence of liver damage, there may not
be excretion of 50 per cent of the load in 4 hours or more.

As in the treatment of edema, the restriction of salt in the
diet will delay the formation of ascites to some extent, although measures directed at improvement of the liver function
are of paramount importance. While repeated paracentesis
leads to protein depletion this is more easily remediable than
the adverse mechanical effects produced by the large accumulation of abdominal fluid, which in itself may lead to increased
salt retention. The moderately lowered serum sodium levels
found in ascitic patients does not respond to administration of
concentrated saline solution, and, if water is also available,
edema increases with the original levels again being obtained.
Salt restriction should be carried out and must ordinarily be
continued for a period of about 6 months in those individuals
who will eventually recover, after which the renal sodium
excretion becomes normal. Mercurial diuresis is of some advantage, but may lead to salt depletion and to potassium depletion as described in Chapter 10.

The author has had occasion to observe several patients
with advanced cirrhosis, in whom the diagnosis of hepatic
coma had been made. These patients presented the picture
of marked lethargy, weakness, confusion and anorexia, and
in each the symptom complex developed either after paracentesis or after only two injections of a mercurial diuretic. Intravenous administration of hypertonic saline produced prompt
and dramatic improvement, thus proving the presence of a
salt depletion syndrome rather than hepatic coma. Serum
sodium levels as low as 126 mEq./L. were found.

TOXEMIAS OF PREGNANCY

There is still considerable difference of opinion as to what
constitutes the clinical picture of pre-eclampsia and eclampsia.
The combination of hypertension, edema and albuminuria
which first make their appearance after the 24th week of
pregnancy, or later, constitute the triad identifying the toxe-

mias. These are frequently confused with a similar symptomatology in patients with kidney disease or hypertension which may worsen during pregnancy and produce an identical picture. Actually these prior nephritics or hypertensives comprise the largest per cent of pregnancy patients with edema, but they are not truly toxemias of pregnancy. Also some patients have difficulty in excreting salt with resulting edema, but without the other evidences of toxemia. Dieckmann terms these "pseudopre-eclampsias." The edema in these patients is controllable by the simple expedient of salt restriction. The blood pressure in normal pregnancy commonly drops to subnormal levels so that an elevation to levels over 130/85 in a pregnant woman can be considered definitely abnormal and suggestive of toxemia.

There is no common agreement as to what represents the pathognomonic structural changes. It is difficult, therefore, to place the site of origin of primary damage or the cause of the clinical picture. Generally speaking, the clinical manifestations most nearly resemble an acute nephritis, although liver necrosis, cerebral damage and other pathology have been described.

BLOOD CHEMICAL CHANGES

Serum sodium and bicarbonate are usually depressed by 5 to 8 mEq., but, since this same change is found in normal pregnancy, it can have no significance as far as toxemia is concerned. Serum pH is within the usual range or at upper limits of normal. Potassium levels are likewise unaltered as are also those of magnesium. Since the blood urea nitrogen levels are usually at the lower limits of normal in pregnancy, elevation of BUN to the upper normal range, which is often found in toxemia, actually represents an elevation and retention of nitrogenous end products. Albumin levels may be somewhat low as in normal pregnancy, although not necessarily. The globulin fraction is often unaltered or even elevated, with this being cited as evidence indicating that hemodilution is not a factor in the hypoalbuminemia. Dieckmann does not believe that hypoproteinemia is a causative factor of the edema, although Strauss believes it may be important in this respect.

The edema of pre-eclampsia and eclampsia, as in the edemas which have already been discussed, comes from abnormal retention of sodium. Whether this is a result primarily of renal damage per se or whether it represents an adrenal response to some other initiating cause is not known. Regardless of the primary cause, the eclamptic patient is not able to excrete a given load of water for over 6 hours, as compared to the normal pregnant patient who diureses in 2 to 4 hours. This would seem to implicate an overproduction of an antidiuretic substance—either of pituitary, liver or placental origin. The depression of serum total base and sodium in toxemia is very likely a manifestation of the tendency to retention of excess water over sodium as seen in other edemas. Peters is of the opinion that the edema is secondary to heart failure and points out the dyspnea, orthopnea and increased venous pressure often found in these patients. Other authors are not in agreement with this and maintain that these are the unusual instances. The terminal episode in toxemia, however, is frequently a circulatory collapse, precipitated by some dehydrating episode such as severe vomiting.

TREATMENT

Aside from the purely obstetric management, the treatment resolves itself, in large part, to restriction of salt to prevent increasing edema. The use of the nonmercurial diuretics is of value, and the cation exchange resins have also been used with advantage. Following severe vomiting, the loss of excessive amounts of sodium may lead to a drop in blood pressure; this should be promptly treated by blood transfusions and with cautious replacement of salt. Strauss stresses the importance of giving protein liberally to these patients, and this has become the accepted procedure in preventing hypoalbuminemia. The improvement in edema by salt restriction does not result in control of the hypertension and the albuminuria, although these may be improved. The dangers of cardiac failure and cerebral edema largely can be avoided by adequate control of excessive salt and water retention.

Bibliography

GENERAL READING

1. Gamble, J. L.: Chemical Anatomy, Physiology and Pathology of Extracellular Fluid: A Lecture Syllabus. ed. 5, Cambridge, Harvard, 1947.
2. Marriott, H. L.: Water and Salt Depletion, Springfield, Ill., Thomas, 1950.
3. Darrow, D. C., and Pratt, E. L.: Fluid therapy: Relation to tissue composition and the expenditure of water and electrolyte, J.A.M.A. 143:365-373, 432-439, 1950.
4. Peters, J. P.: Water balance in health and disease, pp. 271-346, *in* Duncan, G. G., Diseases of Metabolism, ed. 2, Philadelphia, Saunders, 1947.
5. Newburgh, L. H., and Leaf, A.: Significance of the Body Fluids in Clinical Medicine, Springfield, Ill., Thomas, 1950.
6. Moyer, C. A.: Fluid Balance: A Clinical Manual. Chicago Yr. Bk. Pub., 1952.
7. Robinson, J. R., and McCance, R. A.: Water metabolism, Ann. Rev. Physiol. 14:115-142, 1952.
8. Black, D. A. K.: Body-fluid depletion, Lancet 1:305-311, 353-360, 1953.
8a. Weisberg, H. F.: Water, Electrolytes and Acid-Base Balance, Baltimore, Williams & Wilkins, 1953.

ANATOMY AND PHYSIOLOGY

9. Steele, J. M.: Editorial: Body water, Am. J. Med. 9:141-142, 1950.

10. Levitt, M. F., and Gaudino, M.: Measurement of body water compartments, Am. J. Med. 9:208-215, 1950.

11. Hardy, J. D., and Drabkin, D. L., Measurement of body water: Techniques and practical implications, J.A.M.A. 149:1113-1116, 1952.

12. Hardy, J. D., Sen, P. K., and Drabkin, D. L.: The relation of body fluid compartments to body fat, Surg., Gynec. & Obst. 93:103-106, 1951.

13. Lilienthal, J. L., Jr., Baldwin, D., Robinson, P. K., and Zierler, K. L.: Interrelations of magnesium with potassium, phosphorus and creatine in skeletal muscle of man. Tr. A. Am. Physicians 65:223-229, 1952.

14. Verney, E. B.: Croonian lecture: Antidiuretic hormone and factors which determine its release, Proc. Roy. Soc. Med. London, Series B, 135:25-106, 1947.

15. Peters, J. P.: Regulation of the volume and composition of body fluids, J. Missouri M. A. 47:9-17, 1950.

16. ————: Sodium, water and edema, J. Mt. Sinai Hosp. 17:159-175, 1950-51.

17. Smith, H. W.: The excretion of water, Bull. New York Acad. Med. 23:177-195, 1947.

18. Wesson, L. G., Jr., Anslow, W. P., Jr., and Smith, H. W.: The excretion of strong electrolytes, Bull. New York Acad. Med. 24:586-606, 1948.

19. Welt, L. G., Seldin, D. W., Nelson, W. P., III, German, W. J., and Peters, J. P.: Role of the central nervous system in metabolism of electrolytes and water, Arch. Int. Med. 90:355-378, 1952.

20. Leaf, A., and Mamby, A. R.: The normal antidiuretic mechanism in man and dog: Its regulation by extracellular fluid tonicity, J. Clin. Investigation 31:54-59, 1952.

21. Talbot, N. B., Sobel, E. H., McArthur, J. W., and Crawford, J. D.: Functional endocrinology from birth through adolescence, Chap. 8, pp. 497-536, in The Posterior Pituitary, Cambridge, Harvard, 1952.

22. Darrow, D. C., and Yannet, H.: The changes in the distribution of body water accompanying increase and decrease in extracellular electrolyte, J. Clin. Investigation 14:266-275, 1935.

23. Darrow, D. C.: Disturbances of electrolyte metabolism in man and their management. Bull. New York Acad. Med. 24:147-165, 1948.

24. Elkinton, J. R., Winkler, A. W., and Danowski, T. S.: Transfers of cell sodium and potassium in experimental and clinical conditions, J. Clin. Investigation 27:74-81, 1948.

24a. Bergstrom, W. H., and Wallace, W. M.: Bone as a sodium and potassium reservoir, J. Clin. Investigation 33:867-873, 1954.

25. Conn, J. W.: Electrolyte composition of sweat: Clinical implications as an index of adrenal cortical function, Arch. Int. Med. 83:416-428, 1949.

26. Mudge, G. H., Foulks, J., and Gilman, A.: Renal excretion of potassium, Proc. Soc. Exper. Biol. & Med. 67:545-547, 1948.

27. Moore, F. D., and Ball, M. R.: Metabolic Response to Surgery. Springfield, Ill., Thomas, 1952.

28. Heinzen, B. R., Kovach, J. C., and Pifer, M.: Extracellular fluid volume in surgical patients, Surg., Gynec. & Obst. 96:295-298, 1953.

29. Strauss, M. B., Rosenbaum, J. D., and Nelson, W. P., III: Alcohol and homeostasis: The uncompensated water diuresis induced by whiskey, (Abstract). J. Clin. Investigation 28: 813, 1949.

29a. Sieker, H. O., Gaver, O. H., and Henry, J. P.: The effect of negative pressure breathing on water and electrolyte excretion by the human kidney, J. Clin. Investigation 32:572-577, 1954.

See also references: 1, 4, 5, 7, 36, 38, 65, 78, 96, 99, 109, 113, 129.

CLINICAL FLUID BALANCE

30. Fantus, B.: Fluid postoperatively: A statistical study, J.A.M.A. 107:14-17, 1936.

31. Talbott, G. D., and King, W.: A bedside method for semiquantitative sodium analysis, Stanford M. Bull. 10:82-86, 1952.

32. Scribner, B. H., Power, M. H., and Rynearson, E. H.: Bedside management of problems of fluid balance, J.A.M.A. 144:1167-1174, 1950.

33. Scribner, B. H.: Bedside determination of bicarbonate in serum, Proc. Staff Meet., Mayo Clin. 25:641-648, 1950.

34. Statland, H.: A fluid and electrolyte balance service for clinical use, J.A.M.A. 150:771-772, 1952.

SURGERY

35. Peters, J. P.: Structure of the blood in relation to surgical problems, Ann. Surg. 112:490-497, 1940.

36. Winfield, J. M., Fox, C. L., Jr., and Mersheimer, W. L.: Etiologic factors in postoperative salt retention and its prevention, Ann. Surg. 134:626-634, 1951.

37. Moore, F. D.: The low sodium syndromes of surgery, J.A.M.A. 154:379-384, 1954.

38. Hayes, M. A., and Coller, F. A.: The neuroendocrine control of water and electrolyte excretion during surgical anesthesia, Surg., Gynec. & Obst. 95:142-149, 1952.

39. Moore, F. D.: Supportive treatment to needs of the surgical patient, J.A.M.A. 141:646-653, 1949.

40. Lans, H. S., Stein, I. F., and Meyer, K. A.: Diagnosis, treatment and prophylaxis of potassium deficiency in surgical patients, Surg., Gynec. & Obst. 95:321-330, 1952.

41. Berry, R. E. L., Iob, V., and Campbell, K. N.: Potassium metabolism in the immediate postoperative period, Arch. Surg. 57:470-478, 1948.

42. Eliel, L. P., Pearson, O. H., and Rawson, R. W.: Postoperative potassium deficit and metabolic alkalosis, New England J. Med. 243:471-478, 518-524, 1950.

43. Elman, R., Shatz, B. A., Keating, R. E., and Weichselbaum, T. E.: Intracellular and extracellular potassium deficits in surgical patients, Ann. Surg. 136:111-131, 1952.

44. Randall, H. T., Habif, D. V., Lockwood, J. S., and Werner, S. C.: Potassium deficiency in surgical patients, Surgery 26:341-363, 1949.

45. Cooke, R. E., and Crowley, L. G.: Replacement of gastric and intestinal fluid losses in surgery, New England J. Med. 246:637-641, 1952.

46. Moore, F. D.: Bodily changes in surgical convalescence, Ann. Surg. 137:289-315, 1953.

47. Aronstam, E., Schmidt, C. H., and Jenkins, E.: Body fluid shifts, sodium and potassium metabolism in patients undergoing thoracic surgical procedures, Ann. Surg. 137:316-324, 1953.

See also references: 3, 6, 27, 28, 31-34, 49, 64, 68, 106, 107.

SALT AND WATER DEPLETION

48. Danowski, T. S.: Newer concepts of the role of sodium in disease, Am. J. Med. 10:468-480, 1951.

49. Maddock, W. G., and Coller, F. A.: Sodium chloride metabolism of surgical patients, Ann. Surg. 112:520-529, 1940.

50. McCance, R. A.: Medical problems in mineral metabolism; III, Experimental human salt deficiency, Lancet 1:823-830, 1936.

51. Leiter, L., Weston, R. E., and Grossman, J.: The low sodium syndrome: Its origin and varieties, Bull. New York Acad. Med. 29:833-845, 1953.

52. Ladell, W. S. S., Waterlow, J. C., and Hudson, M. F.: Desert climate: Physiological and clinical observations, Lancet **2**: 491-496, 1944.
53. Sims, E. A. H., Welt, L. G., Orloff, J., and Needham, J. W.: Asymptomatic hyponatremia in pulmonary tuberculosis, J. Clin. Investigation **29**:1545-1557, 1950.
54. Nadal, J. W., Pedersen, S., and Maddock, W. G.: Comparison between dehydration from salt loss and from water deprivation, J. Clin. Investigation **20**:691-703, 1941.
55. Elkinton, J. R., and Taffel, M.: Prolonged water deprivation in the dog, J. Clin. Investigation **21**:787-794, 1942.
56. Coller, F. A., and Maddock, W. G.: A study of dehydration in humans, Ann. Surg. **102**:947-960, 1935.
57. Winkler, A. W., Danowski, T. S., Elkinton, J. R., and Peters, J. P.: Electrolyte and fluid studies during water deprivation and starvation in human subjects, and the effect of ingestion of fish, of carbohydrate, and of salt solutions, J. Clin. Investigation **23**:807-815, 1944.
58. Hopper, J., Jr., Elkinton, J. R., and Winkler, A. W.: Plasma volume of dogs in dehydration with and without salt loss, J. Clin. Investigation **23**:111-117, 1944.
59. Winkler, A. W., Elkinton, J. R., Hopper, J., Jr., and Hoff, H. E.: Experimental hypertonicity: Alterations in the distribution of body water and the cause of death. J. Clin. Investigation **23**:103-109, 1944.
60. Di Sant'Agnese, P. A., Darling, R. C., Perera, G. A., and Shea, E.: Sweat electrolyte disturbances associated with childhood pancreatic disease, Am. J. Med. **15**:777-784, 1953.
61. Cooper, I. S., and Crevier, P. H.: Neurogenic hypernatremia and hyperchloremia, J. Clin. Endocrinol. **12**:821-829, 1952.

See also references: 2, 6, 8, 22, 37, 45, 67, 90, 91, 112, 115, 121

POTASSIUM AND MAGNESIUM IMBALANCE

62. Mudge, G. H.: Potassium imbalance, Bull. New York Acad. Med. **29**:846-864, 1953.
63. Tarail, R., and Elkinton, J. R.: Potassium deficiency and the role of the kidney in its production, J. Clin. Investigation **28**: 99-113, 1949.
64. Streeten, D. H. P., and Ward-McQuaid, J. N.: Relation of electrolyte changes and adrenocortical activity to paralytic ileus, Brit. M. J. **2**:587-592, 1952.
65. Hoffman, W. S.: Clinical physiology of potassium, J.A.M.A. **144**:1157-1162, 1950.
66. Danowski, T. S.: Newer concepts of the role of potassium in disease, Am. J. Med. **7**:525-531, 1949.

67. Elkinton, J. R., and Winkler, A. W.: Transfers of intracellular potassium in experimental dehydration, J. Clin. Investigation 23:93-101, 1944.

68. Winter, H. A., Hoff, H. E., and Dso, L.: Effect of potassium deficiency upon gastrointestinal motility, Federation Proc. 8: 169, 1949.

69. Engel, F. L., Martin, S. P., and Taylor, H.: On the relation of potassium to the neurological manifestations of hypocalcemic tetany, Bull. Johns Hopkins Hosp. 84:285-301, 1949.

70. Schwartz, W. B., and Relman, A. S.: Metabolic and renal studies in chronic potassium depletion resulting from overuse of laxatives, J. Clin. Investigation 32:258-271, 1953.

71. Surawicz, B., and Lepeschkin, E.: The electrocardiographic pattern of hypopotassemia with and without hypocalcemia, Circulation 8:801-828, 1953.

71a. Tibbetts, D. M., and Aub, J. C.: Magnesium metabolism in health and disease, I. The magnesium and calcium excretion in normal individuals, also the effects of magnesium, chloride and phosphate ions. J. Clin. Investigation 16:491-501, 1937.

71b. Flink, E. B., Stutzman, F. L., Anderson, A. R., Konig, T., and Fraser, R.: Magnesium deficiency after prolonged parenteral fluid administration and after chronic alcoholism complicated by delirium tremens, J. Lab. & Clin. Med. 43:169-183, 1954.

71c. Haynes, B. W., Jr., Crawford, E. S., and DeBakey, M. E.: Magnesium metabolism in surgical patients, Ann. Surg. 136: 659-667, 1952.

71d. Martin, H. E., Mehl, J., and Wertman, M.: Clinical studies of magnesium metabolism, M. Clin. North America 36:1157-1171, 1952.

See also references: 23, 40, 41, 43, 44, 114.

ACID-BASE BALANCE

72. Pitts, R. F.: Acid-base regulation by the kidneys, Am. J. Med. 9:356-372, 1950.

73. Dorman, P. J., Sullivan, W. T., and Pitts, R. F.: The renal response to acute respiratory acidosis, J. Clin. Investigation 33:82-90, 1954.

74. Richards, D. W., Jr.: Inhalational therapy in cardiac diseases and cardiac failure, Bull. New York Acad. Med. 26:384-394, 1950.

75. Gray, J. S.: Pulmonary Ventilation and its Physiological Regulation, pp. 29-46, Springfield, Ill., Thomas, 1950.

76. Comroe, J. H., Jr., and Dripps, R. D.: Physiologic Basis for Oxygen Therapy, pp. 51-52, 58-75, Springfield, Ill., Thomas, 1950.

77. Hartmann, A. F.: Round table discussion: Acidosis and alkalosis, Pediatrics **2**:584-608, 1948.
78. Darrow, D. C., Schwartz, R., Iannucci, J. F., and Coville, F.: Relation of serum bicarbonate concentration to muscle composition, J. Clin. Investigation **27**:198-208, 1948.
79. Orloff, J., Kennedy, T. J., Jr., and Berliner, R. W.: Effect of potassium in nephrectomized rats with hypokolemic alkalosis. J. Clin. Investigation **32**:538-542, 1953.
80. Cooke, R. E., Coughlin, F. R., Jr., Segar, W. E., and Coville, F.: Muscle composition in respiratory acidosis, J. Clin. Investigation **31**:1006-1010, 1952.
81. Cooke, R. E., Segar, W. E., Cheek, D. B., Coville, F. E., and Darrow, D. C.: The extrarenal correction of alkalosis associated with potassium deficiency, J. Clin. Investigation **31**:798-805, 1952.
82. Elkinton, J. R., Squires, R. D., and Singer, R. B.: Intracellular cation exchanges in acidosis due to renal insufficiency; Effects of alkali therapy, J. Clin. Investigation **30**:381-387, 1951.
83. Nadell, J., and Kalinsky, H.: Effects of carbonic anhydrase inhibitor "6063" on electrolytes and acid-base balance in two normal subjects and two patients with respiratory acidosis, J. Clin. Investigation **32**:622-629, 1953.

See also references: 1, 3, 4, 8a, 24, 35, 42, 67.

TREATMENT OF THE DEPLETIONS; ELECTROLYTE SOLUTIONS

84. Mudge, J. H.: Introduction to a symposium on electrolyte metabolism, Am. J. Med. **15**:761-764, 1953.
85. Butler, A. M., and Talbot, N. B.: I, Estimation and provision of daily maintenance requirements, New England J. Med. **231**:585-590, 1944.
86. ————: Medical progress: Parenteral-fluid therapy; II, The estimation of losses incident to starvation and dehydration with acidosis or alkalosis and the provision of repair therapy, New England J. Med. **231**:621-628, 1944.
87. Mann, G. V., and Stare: F. J.: Nutritional needs in illness and disease, J.A.M.A. **142**:409-419, 1950.
88. Elkinton, J. R., and Tarail, R.: The present status of potassium therapy, Am. J. Med. **9**:200-207, 1950.
89. Howard, J. E., and Carey, R. A.: The use of potassium in therapy, J. Clin. Endocrinol. **9**:691-713, 1949.
90. Abbott, W. E., Levey, S., Foreman, R. C., Krieger, H., and Holden, W. D.: Danger of administering parenteral fluids by hypodermoclysis, Surgery **32**:305-315, 1952.
91. Editorial: Administration of fluids by hypodermoclysis, J.A. M.A. **150**:942-943, 1952.

92. Kremen, A. J.: Editorial: Notes on the management of fluid balance, Surgery 32:875-876, 1952.
93. Fox, C. L., Jr., Winfield, J. M., Slobody, L. B., Swindler, C. M., and Lattimer, J. K.: Electrolyte solution approximating plasma concentrations, with increased potassium for routine fluid and electrolyte replacement, J.A.M.A. 148:827-833, 1952.
94. Elman, R., and Weichselbaum, T. E.: Pre- and postoperative parenteral maintenance of electrolyte balance with a salt mixture containing sodium, potassium chloride and phosphate, Ann. Surg. 135:164-172, 1952.
95. Ravdin, I. S.: Plasma Expanders, J.A.M.A. 150:10-13, 1952.
See also references: 2, 3, 6, 8a, 15, 39, 45, 59, 77.

EDEMA, DIURETICS AND WATER INTOXICATION

96. Wood, E. H.: Physiologic mechanisms for preventing edema of the lower extremities, Proc. Staff Meet., Mayo Clin. 27: 2-6, 1952.
97. Leaf, A., and Mamby, A. R.: An antidiuretic mechanism not regulated by extracellular fluid tonicity, J. Clin. Investigation 31:60-71, 1952.
98. Stein, M., Schwartz, R., and Mirsky, I. A.: The antidiuretic activity of plasma of patients with hepatic cirrhosis, congestive heart failure, hypertension, and other clinical disorders, J. Clin. Investigation 33:77-81, 1954.
99. Lusk, J. A., Viar, W. N., and Harrison, T. R.: Further studies on the effects of changes in the distribution of extracellular fluid on sodium excretion, Circulation 6:911-918, 1952.
100. Schwartz, W. B., and Wallace, W. M.: Electrolyte equilibrium during mercurial diuresis, J. Clin. Investigation 30:1089-1104, 1951.
101. Schwartz, W. B.: Role of electrolyte balance in response to mercurial diuretics in congestive heart failure, Bull. New England M. Center 12:213-223, 1950.
102. Greenman, L., Shaler, J. B., and Danowski, T. S.: Biochemical disturbances and clinical symptoms during prolonged exchange resin therapy in congestive heart failure, Am. J. Med. 14:391-403, 1953.
103. Friedberg, C. K., Taymor, R., Minor, J. B., and Halpern, M.: Use of Diamox, a carbonic anhydrase inhibitor, as an oral diuretic in patients with congestive heart failure, New England J. Med. 248:883-889, 1953.
103a. Kolff, W. J., and Leonards, J. R.: Reduction of otherwise intractable edema by dialysis or filtration, Cleveland Clin. Quart. 21:61-71, 1954.

104. Thorn, G. W., and Tyler, F. H.: Clinical management of edema in Bright's disease, M. Clin. North America **31**:1077-1091, 1947.
105. Smyth, F. S., Deamer, W. C., and Phatak, N. M.: Studies in so-called water intoxication, J. Clin. Investigation **12**:55-65, 1933.
106. Helwig, F. C., Schutz, C. B., and Curry, D. E.: Water intoxication: Report of a fatal human case, with clinical pathologic and experimental studies, J.A.M.A. **104**:1569-1575, 1935.
107. Baskin, J. L., Keith, H. M., and Scribner, B. H.: Water metabolism in water intoxication: Review of basic concepts, Am. J. Dis. Child. **83**:618-627, 1953.
See also references: 16, 20, 51, 83, 117.

CARDIAC EDEMA

108. Dock, W.: Congestive heart failure: Adaptation of the body to inadequate cardiac output, J.A.M.A. **140**:1135-1142, 1949.
109. Squires, R. D., Singer, R. B., Moffit, G. R., Jr., and Elkinton, J. R.: Distribution of body fluids in congestive heart failure: II, Abnormalities in serum electrolyte concentration and in acid-base equilibrium, Circulation **4**:697-705, 1951.
110. Squires, R. D., Crosley, A. P., Jr., and Elkinton, J. R.: Distribution of blood plasma in congestive heart failure: III, Exchanges in patients during diuresis, Circulation **4**:868-880, 1951.
111. Elkinton, J. R., Squires, R. D., and Bluemle, L. W., Jr.: Distribution of body fluids in congestive heart failure: IV, Exchanges in patients refractory to mercurial diuretics, treated with sodium and potassium, Circulation **5**:58-73, 1952.
112. Schroeder, H. A.: Renal failure associated with low extracellular sodium chloride; The low salt syndrome, J.A.M.A. **141**:117-124, 1949.
113. Iseri, L. T., McCaughey, R. S., Alexander, L., Boyle, A. J., and Myers, G. B.: Plasma sodium and potassium concentrations in congestive heart failure; Relationship to pathogenesis of failure, Am. J. M. Sc. **224**:135-145, 1952.
114. Friedberg, C. K.: Medical progress: Electrolyte and fluid disturbances in congestive heart failure, New England J. Med. **245**:812-821, 852-859, 1951.
115. Danowski, T. S.: Electrolytes and congestive failure, Ann. Int. Med. **37**:453-464, 1952.
116. Lown, B., Salzberg, H., Enselberg, C. D., and Weston, R. E.: Interrelation between potassium metabolism and digitalis toxicity in heart failure, Proc. Soc. Exper. Biol. & Med. **76**:797-801, 1951.

116a. Laragh, J. H.: The effect of potassium chloride on hypo-natremia, J. Clin. Investigation 33:807-818, 1954.
See also references: 51, 53, 71, 74, 100, 101, 102, 129.

KIDNEY DISEASE

117. Peters, J. P.: Edema of acute nephritis, Am. J. Med. 14:448-458, 1953.
118. Derow, H. A.: Medical progress: Management of acute glomerulonephritis, New England J. Med. 249:144-153, 1953.
119. Schoch, H. K.: Potassium deficiency in chronic renal disease, Arch. Int. Med. 88:20-27, 1951.
120. Brown, M. R., Currens, J. H., and Marchand, J. F.: Muscular paralysis and electrocardiographic abnormalities resulting from potassium loss in chronic nephritis, J.A.M.A. 124:545-549, 1944.
121. Thorn, G. W., Koepf, G. F., and Clinton, M., Jr.: Renal failure simulating adrenocortical insufficiency, New England J. Med. 231:76-85, 1944.
122. Elkinton, J. R., Clark, J. K., Squires, R. D., Bluemle, L. W., Jr., and Crosley, A. P.: Treatment of potassium retention in anuria with cation exchange resins, Am. J. M. Sc. 220:547-552, 1950.
123. Joiner, C. L.: Salt-losing nephritis, Lancet 2:454-458, 1952.
124. Kelley, R. A., and Hill, L. D., III: Acute renal insufficiency and the role of potassium with treatment by intestinal lavage, J. Urol. 66:645-660, 1951.
124a. Stock, R. J.: The conservative management of acute urinary suppression, Bull. New York Acad. Med. 28:507-522, 1952.
124b. Swann, R. C., and Merrill, J. P.: The clinical course of acute renal failure, Medicine 32:215-292, 1953.
125. Ravin, I. S., Aronson, P. B., and Yules, J. H.: Complications of diuretic phase of lower nephron nephrosis, New England J. Med. 244:830-832, 1951.
126. Merrill, J. P.: Medical progress: The artificial kidney, New England J. Med. 246:17-27, 1952.
127. Eiseman, B., and Bricker, E. M.: Electrolyte absorption following bilateral uretero-enterostomy into an isolated intestinal segment, Ann. Surg. 136:761-769, 1952.
128. D'Agostino, A., Leadbetter, W. F., and Schwartz, W. B.: Alterations in the ionic composition of isotonic saline solution instilled into the colon, J. Clin. Investigation 32:444-448, 1953.
129. Bills, C. E., McDonald, F. G., Niedermeier, W., and Schwartz, M. C.: Sodium and potassium in foods and waters, J. Am. Dietet. A. 25:304-314, 1949.
See also references: 1, 4, 5, 17, 18, 26, 34, 63, 72, 104.

DIABETES

130. Seldin, D. W., and Tarail, R.: The metabolism of glucose and electrolytes in diabetic acidosis, J. Clin. Investigation 29: 552, 1950.
131. Howard, J. E.: Observations on the therapy of diabetic acidosis, Proc. Am. Diabetes A. 10:152-160, 1950.
132. Butler, A. M.: Medical progress: Diabetic coma, New England J. Med. 243:648-659, 1950.
133. Sprague, R. G., and Power, M. H.: Electrolyte metabolism in diabetic acidosis, J.A.M.A. 151:970-976, 1953.
134. Peters, J. P.: Diabetic acidosis, Metabolism 1:223-235, 1952.
135. Nadler, C. S., Bellet, S., Gazes, P. C., and Steiger, W. A.: Administration of potassium to patients with prolonged vomiting and diabetic acidosis, J. Lab. & Clin. Med. 35:842-853, 1950.
136. Danowski, T. S., Peters, J. H., Rathbun, J. C., Quashnock, J. M., and Greenman, L.: Studies in diabetic acidosis and coma with particular emphasis on the retention of administered potassium, J. Clin. Investigation 28:1-9, 1949.
137. Perry, S. M., and Rosenbaum, S. L.: Hypopotassemia in untreated diabetic coma, New England J. Med. 245:847-851, 1951.
138. Miller, M., Drucker, W. R., Owens, J. E., Craig, J. W., and Woodward, H., Jr.: Metabolism of intravenous fructose and glucose in normal and diabetic subjects, J. Clin. Investigation 31:115-125, 1952.
139. Darragh, J. H., Womersley, R. A., and Meroney, W. H.: Fructose in the treatment of diabetic ketosis, J. Clin. Investigation 32:1214-1221, 1953.
140. Talbot, N. B., Sobel, E. H., McArthur, J. W., and Crawford, J. D.: The pancreatic islets, *in* Functional Endocrinology from Birth Through Adolescence, Chap. 9, pp. 543-549, Cambridge, Harvard, 1952.

PEDIATRICS

141. Smith, C. A.: The Physiology of the Newborn Infant, pp. 270-295, ed. 2, Springfield, Ill., Thomas, 1951.
142. Graham, B. D., Wilson, J. L., Tsao, M. U., Baumann, M. L., and Brown, S.: Development of neonatal electrolyte homeostasis, Pediatrics 8:68-78, 1951.
143. McCance, R. A.: Renal physiology in infancy, Am. J. Med. 9:229-241, 1950.
144. Gamble, J. L.: Deficits in diarrhea, J. Pediat. 30:488-494, 1947.

145. Darrow, D. C.: Therapeutic measures promoting recovery from the physiologic disturbances of infantile diarrhea, Pediatrics 9:519-533, 1952.
146. Etteldorf, J. N., Hill, F. S., Tuttle, A. H., Pinheiro, D., Bass, A. C., and Overman, R. R.: Alterations in blood chemistry caused by diarrhea during infancy as determined by direct analysis of plasma and erythrocytes, Pediatrics 10:694-701, 1952.

See also references: 1, 3, 90, 91, 132.

BURNS

147. Wallace, A. B.: The treatment of burns, Practitioner 170:109-118, 1953.
148. Cope, O., and Moore, F. D.: Redistribution of body water and the fluid therapy of the burned patient, Ann. Surg. 126:1010-1045, 1947.
149. Quimby, W. C., Jr., and Cope, O.: Blood viscosity and the whole blood therapy of burns, Surgery 32:316-325, 1952.
150. Evans, E. I., Purnell, O. J., Robinette, P. W., Batchelor, A., and Martin, M.: Fluid and electrolyte requirements in severe burns, Ann. Surg. 135:804-817, 1952.
151. Reiss, E., Stirman, J. A., Artz, C. P., Davis, J. H., and Amspacher, W. H.: Fluid and electrolyte balance in burns, J.A.M.A. 152:1309-1313, 1953.

CIRRHOTIC ASCITES

152. Ralli, E. P., and Leslie, S. H.: Role of posterior pituitary in production of ascites associated with cirrhosis of liver, pp. 557-562, *in* Soskin, S.: Progress in Clinical Endocrinology, New York, Grune & Stratton, 1950.
153. Post, J., and Patek, A. J., Jr.: Serum proteins in cirrhosis of the liver; I, Relation to prognosis and to formation of ascites, Arch. Int. Med. 69:67-82, 1942.
154. Schilling, J. A., McCoord, A. B., Clausen, S. W., Troup, S. B., and McKee, F. W.: Experimental ascites: Studies of electrolyte balance in dogs with partial and complete occlusion of the portal vein and of the vena cava above and below the liver, J. Clin. Investigation 31:703-710, 1952.
155. Eisenmenger, W. J.: Role of sodium in the formation and control of ascites in patients with cirrhosis, Ann. Int. Med. 37:261-272, 1952.
156. Hanger, F. M., in combined staff clinic: Mechanism of ascites formation, Am. J. Med. 9:102-113, 1950.

157. Hilton, J. G.: Effects of mercurial diuresis in patients with ascites due to cirrhosis, Am. J. Med. **12**:311-318, 1952.
See also references: 51, 100.

TOXEMIAS OF PREGNANCY

157a. Gray, M. J., and Plentl, A. A.: Variations of the sodium space and the total exchangeable sodium during pregnancy, J. Clin. Investigation **32**:347-353, 1954.
158. Dieckmann, W. J.: The Toxemias of Pregnancy, St. Louis, Mosby, 1952.
159. Strauss, M. B.: Toxemias of pregnancy: Types, etiology and treatment, Am. J. Obstet. & Gynec. **38**:199-213, 1939.
160. Dieckmann, W. J., Smitter, R. C., Horner, E. N., Pottinger, R. E., Rynkiewicz, L., and Lundquist, R.: Etiology of preeclampsia; Eclampsia: III, The effect of oral ingestion of sodium chloride and sodium bicarbonate by patients with toxemia of pregnancy, Am. J. Obstet. & Gynec. **61**:1100-1106, 1952.
161. Chesley, L. C.: Toxemia of pregnancy: A survey, Connecticut M. J. **17**:393-397, 1953.
See also reference: 4.

Index

197